TNM

Classification of Malignant Tumours

UICC International Union Against Cancer

TNM

Classification of Malignant Tumours

Edited by
L.H. Sobin and Ch. Wittekind

Fifth Edition

1997

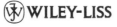 **WILEY-LISS**

A JOHN WILEY & SONS, INC., PUBLICATION

New York • Chichester • Weinheim • Brisbane • Singapore • Toronto

International Union Against Cancer (UICC)
3, rue du Conseil-Général
Ch-1205, Geneva, Switzerland

Editors:
L.H. Sobin, M.D.
Division of Gastrointestinal Pathology
Armed Forces Institute of Pathology
Washington, D.C. 20306, USA

Prof. Dr. med. Ch. Wittekind
Institut für Pathologie der Universität
Liebigstraße 26
D-04103 Leipzig, Germany

Previous English editions were published by the UICC 1968, 1974, 1978, 1987
(with Springer Verlag)

Address All Inquiries to the Publisher
Wiley-Liss, Inc., 605 Third Avenue, New York, NY 10158-0012

Library of Congress Cataloging-in-Publication Data
TNM classification of malignant tumours / edited by L.H. Sobin and Ch. Wittekind.—5th ed.
      p.   cm.
   Includes bibliographical references
   ISBN 0-471-18486-1 (pbk. : alk. paper)
   1. Tumors—classification.   I. Sobin, L. H.   II. Wittekind, Ch. (Christian)   III. International Union against Cancer.
      [DNLM: 1. Neoplasms—classification.   QZ 15 T6255 1997]
   RC258.T583   1997
   616399'4'0012—dc21   97-9162

PRINTED IN THE UNITED STATES OF AMERICA
10   9   8   7   6   5

They are called wise
who put things in their right order
—Thomas Aquinas

CONTENTS

OPHTHALMIC TUMOURS   195

HODGKIN DISEASE   221

NON-HODGKIN LYMPHOMAS   227

PREFACE

In the fifth edition of the TNM Classification most of the tumour sites have remained unchanged from the fourth edition[1] or contain only minor changes, following the basic philosophy of maintaining stability in the classification over time.

The changes and additions reflect new data on prognosis as well as new methods for assessing prognosis.[2] Some of the changes have appeared in the TNM Supplement 1993[3] as proposals. Subsequent support warrants their incorporation into the classification. The major changes are as follows.

- The classification of nasopharyngeal carcinoma has been revised to reflect the needs of radiation oncologists, and in fact is the result of an international collaborative effort with a number of Asian specialists who have great experience with the disease.

---

[1] International Union Against Cancer (UICC): TNM Classification of malignant tumours. 4th ed P. Hermanek, L.H. Sobin (editors). Springer, Berlin Heidelberg New York Tokyo 1987, revised 1992

[2] International Union Against Cancer (UICC): Prognostic Factors in Cancer. P.Hermanek, M.K.Gospodarowicz, D.E. Henson, R.V.P. Hutter, L.H. Sobin (editors) Springer, Berlin Heidelberg New York Tokyo 1995

[3] International Union Against Cancer (UICC): TNM Supplement 1993. A commentary on uniform use. P. Hermanck, D.E. Henson, R.V.P. Hutter, L.H. Sobin (editors) Springer, Berlin Heidelberg New York Tokyo 1993

- The testis tumour classification has been revised to incorporate prognostic serum markers into the stage grouping in a manner that preserves the identity of the anatomic factors while increasing the prognostic value of the classification. It may also serve as a model of how to utilize nonanatomic prognostic factors without obscuring the original building blocks of TNM. It too, was the result of an international study group.

- In a similar manner the new classification of gestational trophoblastic tumours uses hCG levels and duration of disease to modify the anatomic factors in determining the final "stage." It is the result of a FIGO study.

- A new fallopian tube classification is included and is identical with the FIGO classification. Furthermore modifications by FIGO to the vulva and cervix uteri classifications have been adopted in the continuing effort to keep FIGO and TNM classifications identical.

- The classification of brain tumours adopted in the fourth edition (1987) has been deleted in this edition because it has not proved to be particularly useful as a predictor of outcome. Tumour size (T) appears much less important than tumour histology and location. Patient age, function and neurological status, and extent of resection are also considered strong prognostic factors.

- The classification of pediatric tumours has been excluded because of the variety of approaches to these tumours. The classifications used by cooperative research groups are available for those interested in the subject.

- Changes in the classification of urological tumours: prostate, bladder, testis, and kidney, reflect advances in this field and the interest of urological specialists.

As with the fourth edition of TNM, the entire UICC classification—criteria, notation, and stage grouping—is identical to that published by the American Joint Committee on Cancer (AJCC).[4] This is the result of our intent to have only one standard and reflects the collaborative efforts made by all national TNM committees to achieve uniformity in this field.

Changes made between the fourth and fifth edition are indicated by a bar at the left-hand side of the text. To avoid ambiguity, we encourage users to cite the year of the TNM publication they have used in their list of references.

The TNM Prognostic Factors Project welcomes comments from TNM users.

A TNM homepage in the Internet with Frequently Asked Questions and a form for submitting questions or comments on the TNM, Fifth edition can be found at: http://www.uicc.ch/tnm.

International Union Against Cancer (UICC)
3, rue du Conseil-Général
Ch-1205 Geneva, Switzerland
Fax 41 22 8091810

---

[4] AJCC Cancer Staging Manual: I.D. Fleming, J.S. Cooper, D.E. Henson, R.V.P. Hutter, B.J. Kennedy, G.P. Murphy, B. O'Sullivan, J.W. Yarbro (editors) Lippincott, Philadelphia 1997

ACKNOWLEDGEMENTS

The Editors have much pleasure in acknowledging the great help received from the members of the TNM Prognostic Factors Project Committee and the national committees and international organizations listed on pages xix–xxiii.

The fifth edition of the *TNM classification* is the result of a number of consultative editorial meetings organized and supported by the UICC and AJCC secretariates.

The support of the TNM Project by the American Family Insurance Company, Japan, is gratefully acknowledged.

This publication was made possible by grant number R13/CCR012626-01 from the Centers for Disease Control and Prevention (USA). Its contents are solely the responsibility of the authors and do not necessarily represent the official views of the Centers.

ABBREVIATIONS

a	autopsy, p. 12
c	clinical, p. 7
C	certainty factor, p. 12
G	histopathological grading, p. 11
ICD-O	International Classification of Diseases for Oncology, 2nd edition 1990
ICD-O M	morphology rubric of ICD-O
ICD-O T	topography rubric of ICD-O
L	lymphatic invasion, p. 12
m	multiple tumours, pp. 8 and 12
M	distant metastasis
N	regional lymph node metastasis
p	pathological, p. 7
r	recurrent tumour, p. 12
R	residual tumour after treatment, p. 13
T	extent of primary tumour
V	venous invasion, p. 12
y	classification after initial multimodal treatment, p. 11

NATIONAL COMMITTEES
AND INTERNATIONAL
ORGANIZATIONS

AJCC	The American Joint Committee on Cancer
BIJC	The British Isles Joint TNM Classification Committee
CCCS	Canadian Committee on Cancer Staging
CNU - TNM	Comité Nacional Uruguayo TNM
DSK - TNM	Deutschsprachiges TNM-Komitee
EORTC	The European Organization for Research on Treatment of Cancer
FIGO	Fédération Internationale de Gynécologie et d'Obstétrique
FTNM	The French TNM Group
IPSP	The Italian Prognostic System Project
JJC	The Japanese Joint Committee

MEMBERS OF UICC COMMITTEES
ASSOCIATED WITH THE TNM SYSTEM

In 1950 the UICC appointed a *Committee on Tumour Nomenclature and Statistics*. In 1954 this Committee became known as the *Committee on Clinical Stage Classification and Applied Statistics* and in 1966 it was named the *Committee on TNM Classification*. Taking into consideration new factors of prognosis the Committee was named in 1994 the *TNM Prognostic Factor Project Committee*.

The members who have served on these committees are:

Anderson, W.A.D.	USA
Baclesse, F.	France
Badellino, F.	Italy
Barajas-Vallejo, E.	Mexico
Blinov, N.	Russia
Bucalossi, P.	Italy
Burn, I.	United Kingdom
Bush, R.S.	Canada
Carr, D.T.	USA
Copeland, M.M.	USA
Costachel, O.	Romania
Denis, L.	Belgium
Denoix, P.	France
Fischer, A.W.	Federal Republic of Germany

INTRODUCTION

The History of the TNM System

The TNM System for the classification of malignant tumours was developed by Pierre Denoix (France) between the years 1943 and 1952.[1]

In 1950 the UICC appointed a *Committee on Tumour Nomenclature and Statistics* and adopted, as a basis for its work on clinical stage classification, the general definitions of local extension of malignant tumours suggested by the World Health Organization (WHO) Sub-Committee on The Registration of Cases of Cancer as well as Their Statistical Presentation.[2]

In 1953 the Committee held a joint meeting with the International Commission on Stage-Grouping in Cancer and Presentation of the Results of Treatment of Cancer appointed by the International Congress of Radiology. Agreement was reached on a general technique for classification by anatomical extent of the disease, using the TNM system.

In 1954 the Research Commission of the UICC set up a special *Committee on Clinical Stage Classification and Applied Statistics* to "pursue studies in this field and to extend the general technique of classification to cancer at all sites."

[1] P.F. Denoix: Bull Inst Nat Hyg (Paris) 1: 1–69 (1944) and 5–82 (1944)

[2] World Health Organization Technical Report Series, number 53, July 1952, pp. 47–48

In 1958 the Committee published the first recommendations for the clinical stage classification of cancers of the breast and larynx and for the presentation of results.[3]

A second publication in 1959 presented revised proposals for the breast, for clinical use and evaluation over a 5-year period (1960–1964).[4]

Between 1960 and 1967 the Committee published nine brochures describing proposals for the classification of 23 sites. It was recommended that the classification proposals for each site be subjected to prospective or retrospective trial for a 5-year period.

In 1968 these brochures were combined in a booklet, the *Livre de Poche*[5] and a year later, a complementary booklet was published detailing recommendations for the setting-up of field trials, for the presentation of end results and for the determination and expression of cancer survival rates.[6] The *Livre de Poche* was subsequently translated into 11 languages.

In 1974 and 1978, second and third editions[7, 8] were published containing new site classifications and amendments to previously published classifications. The third edition was

[3] International Union Against Cancer (UICC), Committee on Clinical Stage Classification and Applied Statistics: Clinical stage classification and presentation of results, malignant tumours of the breast and larynx. Paris 1958

[4] International Union Against Cancer (UICC), Committee on Stage Classification and Applied Statistics: Clinical stage classification and presentation of results, malignant tumours of the breast. Paris 1959.

[5] International Union Against Cancer (UICC): TNM Classification of malignant tumours. Geneva 1968

[6] International Union Against Cancer (UICC): TNM General Rules. Geneva 1969

[7] International Union Against Cancer (UICC): TNM Classification of malignant tumours. 2nd ed. Geneva 1974

[8] International Union Against Cancer (UICC): TNM Classification of malignant tumours. 3rd ed. M.H. Harmer (editor). Geneva 1978, enlarged and revised 1982

enlarged and revised in 1982. It contained new classifications for selected tumours of childhood. This was carried out in collaboration with La Société Internationale d'Oncologie Pédiatrique (SIOP). A classification of ophthalmic tumours was published separately in 1985.

Over the years some users introduced variations in the rules of classification of certain sites. In order to correct this development, the antithesis of standardization, the national TNM committees in 1982 agreed to formulate a single TNM. A series of meetings was held to unify and update existing classifications as well as to develop new ones. The result was the fourth edition of TNM.[9]

In 1993, the project published the **TNM Supplement.**[10] The purpose of this work was to promote the uniform use of TNM by providing detailed explanations of the TNM rules with practical examples. It also included proposals for new classifications, and optional expansions of selected categories.

In 1995 the project published **Prognostic Factors in Cancer,**[11] a compilation and discussion of prognostic factors in cancer at each of the body sites.

The present (5th) edition contains rules of classification and staging that correspond exactly with those appearing in the

[9] International Union Against Cancer (UICC): TNM Classification of malignant tumours. 4th ed. P.Hermanek, L.H.Sobin (editors). Springer, Berlin Heidelberg New York Tokyo 1987, revised 1992

[10] International Union Against Cancer (UICC): TNM Supplement 1993. A commentary on uniform use. P. Hermanek, D.E. Henson, R.V.P. Hutter, L.H. Sobin (editors) Springer, Berlin Heidelberg New York Tokyo 1993

[11] International Union Against Cancer (UICC): Prognostic factors in cancer. P. Hermanek, M.K. Gospodarowicz, D.E. Henson, R.V.P. Hutter, L.H. Sobin (editors) Springer, Berlin Heidelberg New York Tokyo 1995

fifth edition of the *AJCC Cancer Staging Manual* (1997)[12] and have approval of all national TNM committees. These are listed on pages xix–xxiii together with the names of members of the UICC committees who have been associated with the TNM system.

The UICC recognizes the need for stability in the TNM classification so that data can be accumulated in an orderly way over reasonable periods of time. Accordingly, it is the intention that the classifications published in this booklet should remain unchanged until some major advances in diagnosis or treatment relevant to a particular site require reconsideration of the current classification.

To develop and sustain a classification system acceptable to all requires the closest liaison by all national and international committees. Only in this way will all oncologists be able to use a "common language" in comparing their clinical material and in assessing the results of treatment. The continuing objective of the UICC is to achieve common consent in the classification of anatomical extent of disease.

The Principles of the TNM System

The practice of dividing cancer cases into groups according to so-called stages arose from the fact that survival rates were higher for cases in which the disease was localized than for those in which the disease had extended beyond the organ of origin. These groups were often referred to as early cases and

---

[12] AJCC Cancer Staging Manual: I.D. Fleming, J.S. Cooper, D.E. Henson, R.V.P. Hutter, B.J.Kennedy, G.P. Murphy, B. O'Sullivan, J.W. Yarbro (editors) Lippincott, Philadelphia 1997

late cases, implying some regular progression with time. Actually, the stage of disease at the time of diagnosis may be a reflection not only of the rate of growth and extension of the neoplasm but also of the type of tumour and of the tumour-host relationship.

The staging of cancer is hallowed by tradition, and for the purpose of analysis of groups of patients it is often necessary to use such a method. The UICC believes that it is important to reach agreement on the recording of accurate information on the extent of the disease for each site, because the precise clinical description of malignant neoplasms and histopathological classification (when possible) may serve a number of related objectives, namely

1. To aid the clinician in the planning of treatment
2. To give some indication of prognosis
3. To assist in evaluation of the results of treatment
4. To facilitate the exchange of information between treatment centres
5. To contribute to the continuing investigation of human cancer

The principal purpose to be served by international agreement on the classification of cancer cases by extent of disease is to provide a method of conveying clinical experience to others without ambiguity.

There are many bases or axes of tumour classification: for example, the anatomical site and the clinical and pathological extent of disease, the reported duration of symptoms or signs, the gender and age of the patient, and the histological type and grade. All of these bases or axes represent variables which are known to have an influence on the outcome of the disease. Classification by anatomical extent of disease as determined clinically and histopathologically (when possible) is the one with which the TNM system primarily deals.

The clinician's immediate task is to make a judgment as to prognosis and a decision as to the most effective course of treatment. This judgment and this decision require, among other things, an objective assessment of the anatomical extent of the disease. In accomplishing this, the trend is away from "staging" to meaningful description, with or without some form of summarization.

To meet the stated objectives we need a system of classification

1. Whose basic principles are applicable to all sites regardless of treatment; and
2. Which may be supplemented later by information which becomes available from histopathology and/or surgery.

The TNM system meets these requirements.

The General Rules of the TNM System

The TNM system for describing the anatomical extent of disease is based on the assessment of three components:

  T –   The extent of the primary tumour
  N –   The absence or presence and extent of regional lymph node metastasis
  M –   The absence or presence of distant metastasis.

The addition of numbers to these three components indicates the extent of the malignant disease, thus:

    T0, T1, T2, T3, T4   N0, N1, N2, N3   M0, M1

In effect the system is a "shorthand notation" for describing the extent of a particular malignant tumour.

The general rules applicable to all sites are as follows:

1. All cases should be confirmed microscopically. Any cases not so proved must be reported separately.
2. Two classifications are described for each site, namely:
   (a) *Clinical classification* (Pre-treatment clinical classification), designated **TNM** (or cTNM). This is based on evidence acquired before treatment. Such evidence arises from physical examination, imaging, endoscopy, biopsy, surgical exploration, and other relevant examinations.
   (b) *Pathological classification* (Post-surgical histopathological classification), designated **pTNM.** This is based on the evidence acquired before treatment, supplemented or modified by the additional evidence acquired from surgery and from pathological examination. The pathological assessment of the primary tumour (pT) entails a resection of the primary tumour or biopsy adequate to evaluate the highest pT category. The pathological assessment of the regional lymph nodes (pN) entails removal of nodes adequate to validate the absence of regional lymph node metastasis (pN0) and sufficient to evaluate the highest pN category. The pathological assessment of distant metastasis (pM) entails microscopic examination.
3. After assigning T, N, and M and/or pT, pN, and pM categories, these may be grouped into stages. The TNM classification and stage grouping, once established, must remain unchanged in the medical records. The clinical stage is essential to select and evaluate therapy, while the pathological stage provides the most precise data to estimate prognosis and calculate end results.
4. If there is doubt concerning the correct T, N, or M category to which a particular case should be allotted, then the

lower (i.e., less advanced) category should be chosen. This will also be reflected in the stage grouping.

5. In the case of multiple simultaneous tumours in one organ, the tumour with the highest T category should be classified and the multiplicity or the number of tumours should be indicated in parentheses, e.g., T2 (m) or T2 (5). In simultaneous bilateral cancers of paired organs, each tumour should be classified independently. In tumours of the thyroid, liver, fallopian tube, and ovary, multiplicity is a criterion of T classification.

6. Definitions of TNM categories and stage grouping may be telescoped or expanded for clinical or research purposes as long as basic definitions recommended are not changed. For instance, any T, N, or M can be divided into subgroups.

Anatomical Regions and Sites

The sites in this classification are listed by code number of the International Classification of Diseases for Oncology (ICD-0, 2nd edition, World Health Organization, Geneva, 1990).

Each region or site is described under the following headings:

- Rules for classification with the procedures for assessing the T, N, and M categories
- Anatomical sites, and subsites if appropriate
- Definition of the regional lymph nodes
- TNM Clinical classification
- pTNM Pathological classification
- G Histopathological grading
- Stage grouping
- Summary for the region or site

TNM Clinical Classification

The following general definitions are used throughout:

T – Primary Tumour

TX   Primary tumour cannot be assessed
T0   No evidence of primary tumour
Tis Carcinoma in situ
T1, T2, T3, T4   Increasing size and/or local extent of the
        primary tumour

N – Regional Lymph Nodes

NX   Regional lymph nodes cannot be assessed
N0   No regional lymph node metastasis
N1, N2, N3   Increasing involvement of regional lymph
        nodes

Notes: Direct extension of the primary tumour into lymph nodes is classified as
        lymph node metastasis. Metastasis in any lymph node other than regional is
        classified as a distant metastasis.

M – Distant Metastasis

MX   Distant metastasis cannot be assessed
M0   No distant metastasis
M1   Distant metastasis

The category M1 may be further specified according to the
following notation:

Pulmonary	PUL	(C34)	Bone marrow	MAR	(C42.1)
Osseous	OSS	(C40,41)	Pleura	PLE	(C38.4)
Hepatic	HEP	(C22)	Peritoneum	PER	(C48.1,2)
Brain	BRA	(C71)	Adrenals	ADR	(C74)
Lymph nodes	LYM	(C77)	Skin	SKI	(C44)
Others	OTH				

Subdivisions of TNM

Subdivisions of some main categories are available for those who need greater specificity (e.g., T1a, 1b or N2a, 2b).

pTNM Pathological Classification

The following general definitions are used throughout:

pT – Primary Tumour

pTX Primary tumour cannot be assessed histologically
pT0 No histological evidence of primary tumour
pTis Carcinoma in situ
pT1, pT2, pT3, pT4   Increasing size and/or local extent of the primary tumour histologically

pN – Regional Lymph Nodes

pNX Regional lymph nodes cannot be assessed histologically
pN0 No regional lymph node metastasis histologically
pN1, pN2, pN3   Increasing involvement of regional lymph nodes histologically

Notes: Direct extension of the primary tumour into lymph nodes is classified as lymph node metastasis.
A tumour nodule greater than 3 mm in the connective tissue of a lymph drainage area without histologic evidence of residual lymph node is classified in the pN category as a regional lymph node metastasis. A tumour nodule of up to 3 mm is classified in the pT category, i.e., discontinuous extension.
When size is a criterion for pN classification, e.g., in breast carcinoma, measurement is made of the metastasis, not of the entire lymph node.

pM – Distant Metastasis

pMX Distant metastasis cannot be assessed microscopically
pM0 No distant metastasis microscopically
pM1 Distant metastasis microscopically

The category pM1 may be further specified in the same way as M1 (see page 9).

Subdivisions of pTNM

Subdivisions of some main categories are available for those who need greater specificity (e.g., pT1a, 1b or pN2a, 2b).

Histopathological Grading

In most sites further information regarding the primary tumour may be recorded under the following heading:

G – Histopathological Grading

    GX   Grade of differentiation cannot be assessed
    G1   Well differentiated
    G2   Moderately differentiated
    G3   Poorly differentiated
    G4   Undifferentiated

Note: Grades 3 and 4 can be combined in some circumstances as "G3–4, Poorly differentiated or undifferentiated."

Additional Descriptors

For identification of special cases in the TNM or pTNM classification, the y, r, a, and m symbols are used. Although they do not affect the stage grouping, they indicate cases needing separate analysis.

y Symbol. In those cases in which classification is performed during or following initial multimodality therapy, the TNM or pTNM categories are identified by a y prefix.

r Symbol. Recurrent tumours, when staged after a disease-free interval, are identified by the prefix r.

a Symbol. The prefix a indicates that classification is first determined at autopsy.

m Symbol. The suffix m, in parentheses, is used to indicate the presence of multiple primary tumours at a single site.

Optional Descriptors

L – Lymphatic Invasion

LX   Lymphatic invasion cannot be assessed
L0   No lymphatic invasion
L1   Lymphatic invasion

V – Venous Invasion

VX   Venous invasion cannot be assessed
V0   No venous invasion
V1   Microscopic venous invasion
V2   Macroscopic venous invasion

Note: Macroscopic involvement of the wall of veins (with no tumour within the veins) is classified as V2.

C-Factor

The C-factor, or certainty factor, reflects the validity of classification according to the diagnostic methods employed. Its use is optional.

The C-factor definitions are:

C1   Evidence from standard diagnostic means (e.g., inspection, palpation, and standard radiography, intraluminal endoscopy for tumours of certain organs)

C2   Evidence obtained by special diagnostic means (e.g., radiographic imaging in special projections, tomography, computerized tomography [CT], ultrasonography, lymphography, angiography; scintigraphy; magnetic resonance imaging [MRI]; endoscopy, biopsy, and cytology)

C3   Evidence from surgical exploration, including biopsy and cytology

C4   Evidence of the extent of disease following definitive surgery and pathological examination of the resected specimen

C5   Evidence from autopsy

Example: Degrees of C may be applied to the T, N, and M categories. A case might be described as T3C2, N2C1, M0C2.

The TNM clinical classification is therefore equivalent to C1, C2, and C3 in varying degrees of certainty, while the pTNM pathological classification generally is equivalent to C4.

Residual Tumour (R) Classification

The absence or presence of residual tumour after treatment is described by the symbol R. Its use is optional.

TNM and pTNM describe the anatomical extent of cancer in general without considering treatment. They can be supplemented by the R classification, which deals with tumour status after treatment. It reflects the effects of therapy, influences further therapeutic procedures and is a strong predictor of prognosis.

The definitions of the R categories are:

RX   Presence of residual tumour cannot be assessed
R0   No residual tumour
R1   Microscopic residual tumour
R2   Macroscopic residual tumour

Stage Grouping

Classification by the TNM system achieves reasonably precise description and recording of the apparent anatomical extent of disease. A tumour with four degrees of T, three degrees of N, and two degrees of M will have 24 TNM categories. For purposes of tabulation and analysis, except in very large series, it is necessary to condense these categories into a convenient number of TNM stage groups.

Carcinoma in situ is categorized stage 0; cases with distant metastasis stage IV (except at certain sites, e.g., papillary and follicular carcinoma of thyroid).

The grouping adopted is such as to ensure, as far as possible, that each group is more or less homogeneous in respect of survival, and that the survival rates of these groups for each cancer site are distinctive.

For pathological stage grouping, if sufficient tissue has been removed for pathologic examination to evaluate the highest T and N categories, M1 may be either clinical (cM1) or pathologic (pM1). However, if only a distant metastasis has had microscopic confirmation, the classification is pathologic (pM1) and the stage is pathologic.

Site Summary

As an aide-mémoire or as a means of reference, a simple summary of the chief points which distinguish the most important categories is added at the end of each site. These abridged definitions are not completely adequate, and the full definitions should always be consulted.

Related Classifications

Since 1958 WHO has been involved in a programme aimed at providing internationally acceptable criteria for the histologic diagnosis of tumours. This has resulted in the *International Histological Classification of Tumours,* which contains, in an illustrated multivolume series, definitions of tumour types and a proposed nomenclature. This is now in a second edition.

The *WHO International Classification of Diseases for Oncology (ICD-O)*[13] is a coding system for neoplasms by topography and morphology and for indicating behaviour (e.g., malignant, benign). This coded nomenclature is identical in the morphology field for neoplasms to the Systematized Nomenclature of Medicine (SNOMED).[14]

In the interest of promoting national and international collaboration in cancer research and specifically of facilitating cooperation in clinical investigations, it is recommended that the *International Histological Classification of Tumours* be used for classification and definition of tumour types and that the ICD-O code be used for storage and retrieval of data.

Substantial changes in the 1997 5th edition compared to the 1992 4th edition second revision are marked by a bar at the left-hand side of the page. The same is true for new classifications of previously unclassified tumours.

---

[13]WHO: International Classification of Diseases for Oncology, 2nd Ed. Geneva, 1990.

[14]College of American Pathologists: Systematized Nomenclature of Medicine, Chicago, 1982.

HEAD AND NECK TUMOURS

Introductory Notes

The following sites are included:

- Lip, Oral cavity
- Pharynx: Oropharynx, Nasopharynx, Hypopharynx
- Larynx
- Maxillary sinus
- Ethmoid sinus
- Salivary glands
- Thyroid gland

Each site is described under the following headings:

- Rules for classification with the procedures for assessing T, N, and M categories; additional methods may be used when they enhance the accuracy of appraisal before treatment
- Anatomical sites and subsites where appropriate
- Definition of the regional lymph nodes
- TNM Clinical classification
- pTNM Pathological classification
- G Histopathological grading
- Stage grouping
- Summary

Regional Lymph Nodes

The definitions of the N categories for all head and neck sites except nasopharynx and thyroid are the same. Midline nodes are considered ipsilateral nodes except in the thyroid.

Distant Metastasis

The definitions of the M categories for all head and neck sites are the same.

The categories M1 and pM1 may be further specified according to the following notation:

Pulmonary	PUL	Bone marrow	MAR
Osseous	OSS	Pleura	PLE
Hepatic	HEP	Peritoneum	PER
Brain	BRA	Adrenals	ADR
Lymph nodes	LYM	Skin	SKI
Others	OTH		

Histopathological Grading

The definitions of the G categories apply to all head and neck sites except thyroid. These are:

G – Histopathological Grading

GX   Grade of differentiation cannot be assessed
G1   Well differentiatcd
G2   Moderately differentiated
G3   Poorly differentiated
G4   Undifferentiated

R Classification

The absence or presence of residual tumour after treatment
may be described by the symbol R. The definitions of the R
classification apply to all head and neck sites These are:

RX   Presence of residual tumour cannot be assessed
R0   No residual tumour
R1   Microscopic residual tumour
R2   Macroscopic residual tumour

Lip and Oral Cavity
(ICD-O C00, C02-C06)

Rules for Classification

The classification applies only to carcinomas of the vermilion surfaces of the lips and of the oral cavity, including those of minor salivary glands. There should be histological confirmation of the disease.

The following are the procedures for assessing T, N, and M categories:

T categories	Physical examination and imaging
N categories	Physical examination and imaging
M categories	Physical examination and imaging

Anatomical Sites and Subsites

Lip
1. External upper lip (vermilion border) (C00.0)
2. External lower lip (vermilion border) (C00.1)
3. Commissures (C00.6)

Oral Cavity
1. Buccal mucosa
    (i)   Mucosa of upper and lower lips (C00.3, 4)
    (ii) Cheek mucosa (C06.0)
    (iii) Retromolar areas (C06.2)
    (iv) Bucco-alveolar sulci, upper and lower (vestibule of mouth) (C06.1)
2. Upper alveolus and gingiva (upper gum) (C03.0)
3. Lower alveolus and gingiva (lower gum) (C03.1)

4. Hard palate (C05.0)
5. Tongue
    (i) Dorsal surface and lateral borders anterior to vallate papillae (anterior two-thirds) (C02.0, 1)
    (ii) Inferior (ventral) surface (C02.2)
6. Floor of mouth (C04)

Regional Lymph Nodes

The regional lymph nodes are the cervical nodes.

TNM Clinical Classification

T – Primary Tumour

TX   Primary tumour cannot be assessed
T0   No evidence of primary tumour
Tis Carcinoma in situ

T1   Tumour 2 cm or less in greatest dimension
T2   Tumour more than 2 cm but not more than 4 cm in greatest dimension
T3   Tumour more than 4 cm in greatest dimension
T4   *Lip:* Tumour invades adjacent structures, e.g., through cortical bone, inferior alveolar nerve, floor of mouth, skin of face.
     Oral Cavity: Tumour invades adjacent structures, e.g., through cortical bone, into deep (extrinsic) muscle of tongue, maxillary sinus, skin. (Superficial erosion alone of bone/tooth socket by gingival primary is not sufficient to classify a tumour as T4.)

N – Regional Lymph Nodes

NX   Regional lymph nodes cannot be assessed

N0   No regional lymph node metastasis

N1   Metastasis in a single ipsilateral lymph node, 3 cm or less in greatest dimension

N2   Metastasis in a single ipsilateral lymph node, more than 3 cm but not more than 6 cm in greatest dimension; or in multiple ipsilateral lymph nodes, none more than 6 cm in greatest dimension; or in bilateral or contralateral lymph nodes, none more than 6 cm in greatest dimension

     N2a   Metastasis in a single ipsilateral lymph node, more than 3 cm but not more than 6 cm in greatest dimension

     N2b   Metastasis in multiple ipsilateral lymph nodes, none more than 6 cm in greatest dimension

     N2c   Metastasis in bilateral or contralateral lymph nodes, none more than 6 cm in greatest dimension

N3   Metastasis in a lymph node more than 6 cm in greatest dimension

Note: Midline nodes are considered ipsilateral nodes.

M – Distant Metastasis

MX   Distant metastasis cannot be assessed

M0   No distant metastasis

M1   Distant metastasis

pTNM Pathological Classification

The pT, pN, and pM categories correspond to the T, N, and M categories.

pN0   Histological examination of a selective neck dissection specimen will ordinarily include 6 or more lymph nodes. Histological examination of a radical or modified radical neck dissection specimen will ordinarily include 10 or more lymph nodes.

G Histopathological Grading

See definitions on page 18

Stage Grouping

Stage 0	Tis	N0	M0
Stage I	T1	N0	M0
Stage II	T2	N0	M0
Stage III	T3	N0	M0
	T1	N1	M0
	T2	N1	M0
	T3	N1	M0
Stage IVA	T4	N0	M0
	T4	N1	M0
	Any T	N2	M0
Stage IVB	Any T	N3	M0
Stage IVC	Any T	Any N	M1

Summary

Lip, Oral Cavity	
T1	≤2 cm
T2	>2 to 4 cm
T3	>4 cm
T4	Adjacent structures
N1	Ipsilateral single ≤3 cm
N2	Ipsilateral single >3 to 6 cm
	Ipsilateral multiple ≤6 cm
	Bilateral, contralateral ≤6 cm
N3	>6 cm

Pharynx
(ICD-O C01, C05.1, 2, C09, C10.0, 2, 3, C11-13)

Rules for Classification

The classification applies only to carcinomas. There should be histological confirmation of the disease.

The following are the procedures for assessing T, N, and M categories:

T categories   Physical examination, endoscopy and imaging
N categories   Physical examination and imaging
M categories   Physical examination and imaging

Anatomical Sites and Subsites

Oropharynx (C01, C05.1, 2, C09.0, 1, 9, C10.0, 2, 3)
  1. Anterior wall (glosso-epiglottic area)
     (i)   Base of tongue (posterior to the vallate papillae or posterior third) (C01)
     (ii) Vallecula (C10.0)
  2. Lateral wall (C10.2)
     (i)   Tonsil (C09.9)
     (ii) Tonsillar fossa (C09.0) and tonsillar (faucial) pillars (C09.1)
     (iii) Glossotonsillar sulci (tonsillar pillars) (C09.1)
  3. Posterior wall (C10.3)
  4. Superior wall
     (i)   Inferior surface of soft palate (C05.1)
     (ii) Uvula (C05.2)

Nasopharynx (C11)

1. Postero-superior wall: extends from the level of the junction of the hard and soft palates to the base of the skull (C11.0, 1)
2. Lateral wall: including the fossa of Rosenmüller (C11.2)
3. Inferior wall: consists of the superior surface of the soft palate (C11.3)

Note: The margin of the choanal orifices, including the posterior margin of the nasal septum, is included with the nasal fossa.

Hypopharynx (C12, C13)

1. Pharyngo-oesophageal junction (postcricoid area) (C13.0): extends from the level of the arytenoid cartilages and connecting folds to the inferior border of the cricoid cartilage, thus forming the anterior wall of the hypopharynx
2. Piriform sinus (C12.9): extends from the pharyngo-epiglottic fold to the upper end of the oesophagus. It is bounded laterally by the thyroid cartilage and medially by the hypopharyngeal surface of the aryepiglottic fold (C13.1) and the arytenoid and cricoid cartilages
3. Posterior pharyngeal wall (C13.2): extends from the superior level of the hyoid bone (or floor of the vallecula) to the level of the inferior border of the cricoid cartilage and from the apex of one piriform sinus to the other

Regional Lymph Nodes

The regional lymph nodes are the cervical nodes.

TNM Clinical Classification

T – Primary Tumour

TX   Primary tumour cannot be assessed
T0   No evidence of primary tumour
Tis   Carcinoma in situ

Oropharynx

T1   Tumour 2 cm or less in greatest dimension
T2   Tumour more than 2 cm but not more than 4 cm in greatest dimension
T3   Tumour more than 4 cm in greatest dimension
T4   Tumour invades adjacent structures, e.g., pterygoid muscles, mandible, hard palate, deep muscle of tongue, larynx

Nasopharynx

T1   Tumour confined to nasopharynx
T2   Tumour extends to soft tissue of oropharynx and/or nasal fossa

    T2a   without parapharyngeal extension*

    T2b   with parapharyngeal extension*

T3   Tumour invades bony structures and/or paranasal sinuses
T4   Tumour with intracranial extension and/or involvement of cranial nerves, infratemporal fossa, hypopharynx, or orbit

Note: *Parapharyngeal extension denotes postero-lateral infiltration of tumour beyond the pharyngo-basilar fascia.

Hypopharynx

T1   Tumour limited to one subsite of hypopharynx (see page 26) and 2 cm or less in greatest dimension
T2   Tumour invades more than one subsite of hypopharynx or an adjacent site, or measures more than 2 cm

but not more than 4 cm in greatest dimension, *without* fixation of hemilarynx

T3   Tumour measures more than 4 cm in greatest dimension, or *with* fixation of hemilarynx

T4   Tumour invades adjacent structures, e.g., thyroid/cricoid cartilage, carotid artery, soft tissues of neck, prevertebral fascia/muscles, thyroid, and/or oesophagus

N – Regional Lymph Nodes (*Oro- and Hypopharynx*)

NX   Regional lymph nodes cannot be assessed

N0   No regional lymph node metastasis

N1   Metastasis in a single ipsilateral lymph node, 3 cm or less in greatest dimension

N2   Metastasis in a single ipsilateral lymph node, more than 3 cm but not more than 6 cm in greatest dimension; or in multiple ipsilateral lymph nodes, none more than 6 cm in greatest dimension; or in bilateral or contralateral lymph nodes, none more than 6 cm in greatest dimension

   N2a   Metastasis in a single ipsilateral lymph node, more than 3 cm but not more than 6 cm in greatest dimension

   N2b   Metastasis in multiple ipsilateral lymph nodes, none more than 6 cm in greatest dimension

   N2c   Metastasis in bilateral or contralateral lymph nodes, none more than 6 cm in greatest dimension

N3   Metastasis in a lymph node more than 6 cm in greatest dimension

Note: Midline nodes are considered ipsilateral nodes.

N – Regional Lymph Nodes *(Nasopharynx)*

NX   Regional lymph nodes cannot be assessed
N0   No regional lymph node metastasis
N1   Unilateral metastasis in lymph node(s), 6 cm or less in greatest dimension, above supraclavicular fossa
N2   Bilateral metastasis in lymph node(s), 6 cm or less in greatest dimension, above supraclavicular fossa
N3   Metastasis in lymph node(s)
      (a) greater than 6 cm in dimension
      (b) in the supraclavicular fossa

Note: Midline nodes are considered ipsilateral nodes.

M – Distant Metastasis

MX   Distant metastasis cannot be assessed
M0   No distant metastasis
M1   Distant metastasis

pTNM Pathological Classification

The pT, pN, and pM categories correspond to the T, N, and M categories.

pN0 Histological examination of a selective neck dissection specimen will ordinarily include 6 or more lymph nodes. Histological examination of a radical or modified radical neck dissection specimen will ordinarily include 10 or more lymph nodes.

G Histopathological Grading

See definitions on page 18.

Stage Grouping (*Oropharynx and Hypopharynx*)

Stage 0	Tis	N0	M0
Stage I	T1	N0	M0
Stage II	T2	N0	M0
Stage III	T1	N1	M0
	T2	N1	M0
	T3	N0, N1	M0
Stage IVA	T4	N0, N1	M0
	Any T	N2	M0
Stage IVB	Any T	N3	M0
Stage IVC	Any T	Any N	M1

Stage Grouping (*Nasopharynx*)

Stage 0	Tis	N0	M0
Stage I	T1	N0	M0
Stage IIA	T2a	N0	M0
Stage IIB	T1	N1	M0
	T2a	N1	M0
	T2b	N0, N1	M0
Stage III	T1	N2	M0
	T2a, T2b	N2	M0
	T3	N0, N1, N2	M0
Stage IVA	T4	N0, N1, N2	M0
Stage IVB	Any T	N3	M0
Stage IVC	Any T	Any N	M1

Summary

Pharynx	
	Oropharynx
T1	≤2 cm
T2	>2 to 4 cm
T3	>4 cm
T4	Invades adjacent structures
	Hypopharynx
T1	≤2 cm and limited to one subsite
T2	>2 to 4 cm or more than one subsite
T3	>4 cm or with larynx fixation
T4	Invades adjacent structures
	Oropharynx and Hypopharynx
N1	Ipsilateral single ≤3 cm
N2	Ipsilateral single >3 to 6 cm
	Ipsilateral multiple ≤6 cm
	Bilateral, contralateral ≤6 cm
N3	>6 cm

Nasopharynx	
T1	Nasopharynx
T2	Soft tissue of oropharynx and/or nasal fossa
T2a	Without parapharyngeal extension
T2b	With parapharyngeal extension
T3	Invades bony structures and/or paranasal sinuses
T4	Intracranial extension, involvement of cranial nerves, infratemporal fossa, hypopharynx, orbit
N1	Unilateral metastasis in lymph node(s) ≤6 cm, above supraclavicular fossa
N2	Bilateral metastasis in lymph node(s) ≤6 cm, above supraclavicular fossa
N3	(a) >6 cm (b) in the supraclavicular fossa

Larynx
(ICD-O C32.0, 1, 2, C10.1)

Rules for Classification

The classification applies only to carcinomas. There should be histological confirmation of the disease.

The following are the procedures for assessing T, N, and M categories:

T categories	Physical examination, laryngoscopy, and imaging
N categories	Physical examination and imaging
M categories	Physical examination and imaging

Anatomical Sites and Subsites

1. Supraglottis (C32.1)
    - (i) Suprahyoid epiglottis [including tip, lingual (anterior) (C10.1), and laryngeal surfaces] — *Epilarynx (including marginal zone)*
    - (ii) Aryepiglottic fold, laryngeal aspect
    - (iii) Arytenoid
    - (iv) Infrahyoid epiglottis — *Supraglottis excluding epilarynx*
    - (v) Ventricular bands (false cords)
2. Glottis (C32.0)
    - (i) Vocal cords
    - (ii) Anterior commissure
    - (iii) Posterior commissure
3. Subglottis (C32.2)

Regional Lymph Nodes

The regional lymph nodes are the cervical nodes.

TNM Clinical Classification

T – Primary Tumour

TX   Primary tumour cannot be assessed
T0   No evidence of primary tumour
Tis   Carcinoma in situ

Supraglottis

T1   Tumour limited to one subsite of supraglottis with normal vocal cord mobility
T2   Tumour invades mucosa of more than one adjacent subsite of supraglottis or glottis or region outside the supraglottis (e.g., mucosa of base of tongue, vallecula, medial wall of piriform sinus) without fixation of the larynx
T3   Tumour limited to larynx with vocal cord fixation and/or invades any of the following: postcricoid area, pre-epiglottic tissues, deep base of tongue
T4   Tumour invades through thyroid cartilage, and/or extends into soft tissues of the neck, thyroid, and/or oesophagus

Glottis

T1   Tumour limited to vocal cord(s) (may involve anterior or posterior commissure) with normal mobility
        T1a   Tumour limited to one vocal cord
        T1b   Tumour involves both vocal cords
T2   Tumour extends to supraglottis and/or subglottis, and/or with impaired vocal cord mobility
T3   Tumour limited to larynx with vocal cord fixation

T4   Tumour invades through thyroid cartilage and/or extends to other tissues beyond the larynx, e.g., trachea, soft tissues of neck, thyroid, pharynx

Subglottis
T1   Tumour limited to subglottis
T2   Tumour extends to vocal cord(s) with normal or impaired mobility
T3   Tumour limited to larynx with vocal cord fixation
T4   Tumour invades through cricoid or thyroid cartilage and/or extends into other tissues beyond the larynx, e.g., trachea, soft tissues of neck, thyroid, oesophagus

N – Regional Lymph Nodes
NX   Regional lymph nodes cannot be assessed
N0   No regional lymph nodes
N1   Metastasis in a single ipsilateral lymph node, 3 cm or less in greatest dimension
N2   Metastasis in a single ipsilateral lymph node, more than 3 cm but not more than 6 cm in greatest dimension; or in multiple ipsilateral lymph nodes, none more than 6 cm in greatest dimension; or in bilateral or contralateral lymph nodes, none more than 6 cm in greatest dimension
   N2a   Metastasis in a single ipsilateral lymph node, more than 3 cm but not more than 6 cm in greatest dimension
   N2b   Metastasis in multiple ipsilateral lymph nodes, none more than 6 cm in greatest dimension
   N2c   Metastasis in bilateral or contralateral lymph nodes, none more than 6 cm in greatest dimension
N3   Metastasis in a lymph node more than 6 cm in greatest dimension

Note: Midline nodes are considered ipsilateral nodes.

M – Distant Metastasis

MX   Distant metastasis cannot be assessed
M0   No distant metastasis
M1   Distant metastasis

pTNM Pathological Classification

The pT, pN, and pM categories correspond to the T, N, and M categories.

pN0 Histological examination of a selective neck dissection specimen will ordinarily include 6 or more lymph nodes. Histological examination of a radical or modified radical neck dissection specimen will ordinarily include 10 or more lymph nodes.

G Histopathological Grading

See definitions on page 18.

Stage Grouping

Stage 0	Tis	N0	M0
Stage I	T1	N0	M0
Stage II	T2	N0	M0
Stage III	T1	N1	M0
	T2	N1	M0
	T3	N0, N1	M0
Stage IVA	T4	N0	M0
	T4	N1	M0
	Any T	N2	M0
Stage IVB	Any T	N3	M0
Stage IVC	Any T	Any N	M1

Summary

Larynx	
	Supraglottis
T1	One subsite, normal mobility
T2	Involving mucosa of more than one adjacent subsite of supraglottis or glottis or adjacent region outside the supraglottis; without fixation
T3	Limited to larynx with vocal cord fixation or invades postcricoid area, pre-epiglottic tissues, base of tongue
T4	Extends beyond larynx
	Glottis
T1	Limited to vocal cord(s), normal mobility
T2	Supraglottis, subglottis, impaired cord mobility
T3	Cord fixation
T4	Extends beyond larynx
	Subglottis
T1	Limited to the subglottis
T2	Extends to vocal cord(s) with normal/ impaired mobility
T3	Cord fixation
T4	Extends beyond larynx
	All Sites
N1	Ipsilateral single ≤3 cm
N2	Ipsilateral single >3 to 6 cm
	Ipsilateral multiple ≤6 cm
	Bilateral, contralateral ≤6 cm
N3	>6 cm

Paranasal Sinuses
(C31.0, 1)

Rules for Classification

The classification applies only to carcinomas. There should be histological confirmation of the disease.

The following are the procedures for assessing T, N, and M categories:

T categories	Physical examination and imaging
N categories	Physical examination and imaging
M categories	Physical examination and imaging

Anatomical Subsites

- Maxillary sinus (C31.0)
- Ethmoid sinus (C31.1)

Regional Lymph Nodes

The regional lymph nodes are the cervical nodes.

TNM Clinical Classification

T – Primary Tumour

TX	Primary tumour cannot be assessed
T0	No evidence of primary tumour
Tis	Carcinoma in situ

Maxillary Sinus

  T1   Tumour limited to the antral mucosa with no erosion
        or destruction of bone
  T2   Tumour causing bone erosion or destruction, except
        for the posterior antral wall, including extension into
        hard palate and/or middle nasal meatus
  T3   Tumour invades any of the following: bone of poste-
        rior wall of maxillary sinus, subcutaneous tissues,
        skin of cheek, floor or medial wall of orbit,
        infratemporal fossa, pterygoid plates, ethmoid sinuses
  T4   Tumour invades orbital contents beyond the floor or
        medial wall including apex and/or any of the follow-
        ing: cribriform plate, base of skull, nasopharynx,
        sphenoid sinus, frontal sinus

Ethmoid Sinus

  T1   Tumour confined to ethmoid with or without bone
        erosion
  T2   Tumour extends into nasal cavity
  T3   Tumour extends to anterior orbit and/or maxillary
        sinus
  T4   Tumour with intracranial extension, orbital extension
        including apex, involving sphenoid and/or frontal
        sinus and/or skin of nose

N – Regional Lymph Nodes

  NX   Regional lymph nodes cannot be assessed
  N0   No regional lymph nodes
  N1   Metastasis in a single ipsilateral lymph node, 3 cm or
        less in greatest dimension
  N2   Metastasis in a single ipsilateral lymph node, more
        than 3 cm but not more than 6 cm in greatest dimen-
        sion; or in multiple ipsilateral lymph nodes, none
        more than 6 cm in greatest dimension; or in bilateral

or contralateral lymph nodes, none more than 6 cm in greatest dimension

- N2a   Metastasis in a single ipsilateral lymph node, more than 3 cm but not more than 6 cm in greatest dimension
- N2b   Metastasis in multiple ipsilateral lymph nodes, none more than 6 cm in greatest dimension
- N2c   Metastasis in bilateral or contralateral lymph nodes, none more than 6 cm in greatest dimension
- N3   Metastasis in a lymph node more than 6 cm in greatest dimension

Note: Midline nodes are considered ipsilateral nodes.

M – Distant Metastasis

- MX   Distant metastasis cannot be assessed
- M0   No distant metastasis
- M1   Distant metastasis

pTNM Pathological Classification

The pT, pN, and pM categories correspond to the T, N, and M categories.

pN0   Histological examination of a selective neck dissection specimen will ordinarily include 6 or more lymph nodes. Histological examination of a radical or modified radical neck dissection specimen will ordinarily include 10 or more lymph nodes.

G Histopathological Grading

See definitions on page 18

Stage Grouping

Stage 0	Tis	N0	M0
Stage I	T1	N0	M0
Stage II	T2	N0	M0
Stage III	T1	N1	M0
	T2	N1	M0
	T3	N0, N1	M0
Stage IVA	T4	N0, N1	M0
Stage IVB	Any T	N2	M0
	Any T	N3	M0
Stage IVC	Any T	Any N	M1

Summary

Paranasal Sinuses	
Maxillary Sinus	
T1	Antral mucosa
T2	Bone destruction
T3	Posterior wall maxillary sinus, subcutaneous tissues, skin of cheek, floor/medial wall of orbit, infratemporal fossa, pterygoid plates, ethmoid sinus(es)
T4	Orbital contents, cribriform plate, base of skull, nasopharynx, sphenoid, frontal sinus
Ethmoid Sinus	
T1	Ethmoid
T2	Nasal cavity
T3	Anterior orbit, maxillary sinus
T4	Intracranial cavity, orbital apex, sphenoid, frontal sinus, skin of nose
All Sites	
N1	Ipsilateral single ≤3 cm
N2	Ipsilateral single >3 to 6 cm
	Ipsilateral multiple ≤6 cm
	Bilateral, contralateral ≤6 cm
N3	>6 cm

Salivary Glands
(ICD-O C07, C08)

Rules for Classification

The classification applies only to carcinomas of the major salivary glands: parotid (C07.9), submandibular (submaxillary) (C08.0), and sublingual (C08.1) glands. Tumours arising in minor salivary glands (mucus-secreting glands in the lining membrane of the upper aerodigestive tract) are not included in this classification but at their anatomic site of origin, e.g., lip. There should be histological confirmation of the disease.

The following are the procedures for assessing T, N, and M categories:

T categories	Physical examination and imaging
N categories	Physical examination and imaging
M categories	Physical examination and imaging

Regional Lymph Nodes

The regional lymph nodes are the cervical nodes.

TNM Clinical Classification

T – Primary Tumour
    TX   Primary tumour cannot be assessed
    T0   No evidence of primary tumour

T1   Tumour 2 cm or less in greatest dimension without extraparenchymal extension*

T2   Tumour more than 2 cm but not more than 4 cm in greatest dimension without extraparenchymal extension*

T3   Tumour having extraparenchymal extension without seventh nerve involvement and/or more than 4 cm but not more than 6 cm in greatest dimension*

T4   Tumour invades base of skull, seventh nerve, and/or exceeds 6 cm in greatest dimension

Note: *Extraparenchymal extension is clinical or macroscopic evidence of invasion of skin, soft tissues, bone, or nerve.
Microscopic evidence alone does not constitute extraparenchymal extension for classification purposes.

N – Regional Lymph Nodes

NX   Regional lymph nodes cannot be assessed

N0   No regional lymph node metastasis

N1   Metastasis in a single ipsilateral lymph node, 3 cm or less in greatest dimension

N2   Metastasis in a single ipsilateral lymph node, more than 3 cm but not more than 6 cm in greatest dimension, or in multiple ipsilateral lymph nodes, none more than 6 cm in greatest dimension, or in bilateral or contralateral lymph nodes, none more than 6 cm in greatest dimension

    N2a   Metastasis in a single ipsilateral lymph node, more than 3 cm but not more than 6 cm in greatest dimension

    N2b   Metastasis in multiple ipsilateral lymph nodes, none more than 6 cm in greatest dimension

    N2c   Metastasis in bilateral or contralateral lymph nodes, none more than 6 cm in greatest dimension

N3   Metastasis in a lymph node more than 6 cm in greatest dimension

Note: Midline nodes are considered ipsilateral nodes.

M – Distant Metastasis

MX   Distant metastasis cannot be assessed
M0   No distant metastasis
M1   Distant metastasis

pTNM Pathological Classification

The pT, pN, and pM categories correspond to the T, N, and M categories.

pN0 Histological examination of a selective neck dissection specimen will ordinarily include 6 or more lymph nodes. Histological examination of a radical or modified radical neck dissection specimen will ordinarily include 10 or more lymph nodes.

G Histopathological Grading

See definitions on page 18.

Stage Grouping

Stage I	T1	N0	M0
	T2	N0	M0
Stage II	T3	N0	M0
Stage III	T1	N1	M0
	T2	N1	M0
Stage IV	T4	N0	M0
	T3	N1	M0
	T4	N1	M0
	Any T	N2	M0
	Any T	N3	M0
	Any T	Any N	M1

Summary

Salivary Glands	
T1	≤ 2 cm, without extraparenchymal extension
T2	>2 to 4 cm, without extraparenchymal extension
T3	Extraparenchymal extension, and/or >4 to 6 cm
T4	Base of skull, seventh nerve, and/or >6 cm
N1	Ipsilateral single ≤3 cm
N2	Ipsilateral single >3 to 6 cm
	Ipsilateral multiple ≤6 cm
	Bilateral, contralateral ≤6 cm
N3	>6 cm

Thyroid Gland
(ICD-O C73)

Rules for Classification

The classification applies only to carcinomas. There should be microscopic confirmation of the disease and division of cases by histological type.

The following are the procedures for assessing T, N, and M categories:

T categories	Physical examination, endoscopy, and imaging
N categories	Physical examination and imaging
M categories	Physical examination and imaging

Regional Lymph Nodes

The regional lymph nodes are the cervical and upper mediastinal nodes.

TNM Clinical Classification

T – Primary Tumour

TX   Primary tumour cannot be assessed
T0   No evidence of primary tumour

T1   Tumour 1 cm or less in greatest dimension, limited to the thyroid
T2   Tumour more than 1 cm but not more than 4 cm in greatest dimension, limited to the thyroid
T3   Tumour more than 4 cm in greatest dimension, limited to the thyroid

T4   Tumour of any size extending beyond the thyroid capsule

Note: All categories may be subdivided: (a) solitary tumour, (b) multifocal tumour (the largest determines the classification).

N – Regional Lymph Nodes

NX   Regional lymph nodes cannot be assessed
N0   No regional lymph node metastasis
N1   Regional lymph node metastasis
      N1a   Metastasis in ipsilateral cervical lymph node(s)
      N1b   Metastasis in bilateral, midline, or contralateral cervical or mediastinal lymph node(s)

M – Distant Metastasis

MX   Distant metastasis cannot be assessed
M0   No distant metastasis
M1   Distant metastasis

pTNM Pathological Classification

The pT, pN, and pM categories correspond to the T, N, and M categories.

pN0 Histological examination of a selective neck dissection specimen will ordinarily include 6 or more lymph nodes.

Histopathologic Types

The four major histopathologic types are:

- Papillary carcinoma (including those with follicular foci)
- Follicular carcinoma (including so-called Hürthle cell carcinoma)
- Medullary carcinoma
- Undifferentiated (anaplastic) carcinoma

Stage Grouping

Separate stage groupings are recommended for papillary and follicular, medullary, and undifferentiated carcinomas:

Papillary or Follicular

Under 45 years

Stage I	Any T	Any N	M0
Stage II	Any T	Any N	M1

45 years and older

Stage I	T1	N0	M0
Stage II	T2	N0	M0
	T3	N0	M0
Stage III	T4	N0	M0
	Any T	N1	M0
Stage IV	Any T	Any N	M1

Medullary

Stage I	T1	N0	M0
Stage II	T2	N0	M0
	T3	N0	M0
	T4	N0	M0
Stage III	Any T	N1	M0
Stage IV	Any T	Any N	M1

Undifferentiated

Stage IV	Any T	Any N	Any M
	(all cases are stage IV)		

Summary

Thyroid Gland	
T1	≤1 cm
T2	>1 to 4 cm
T3	>4 cm
T4	Extends beyond gland
N1	Regional

DIGESTIVE SYSTEM TUMOURS

Introductory Notes

The following sites are included:

- Oesophagus
- Stomach
- Small Intestine
- Colon and Rectum
- Anal Canal
- Liver
- Gallbladder
- Extrahepatic Bile Ducts
- Ampulla of Vater
- Pancreas

Each site is described under the following headings:

- Rules for classification with the procedures for assessing T, N, and M categories; additional methods may be used when they enhance the accuracy of appraisal before treatment
- Anatomical sites and subsites where appropriate
- Definition of the regional lymph nodes
- TNM Clinical classification
- pTNM Pathological Classification
- G Histopathological grading
- Stage grouping

Regional Lymph Nodes

The number of lymph nodes ordinarily included in a lymphadenectomy specimen is noted at each site. The designation pN0 is usually based on this figure.

Distant Metastasis

The categories M1 and pM1 may be further specified according to the following notation:

Pulmonary	PUL	Bone marrow	MAR
Osseous	OSS	Pleura	PLE
Hepatic	HEP	Peritoneum	PER
Brain	BRA	Adrenals	ADR
Lymph nodes	LYM	Skin	SKI
Others	OTH		

Histopathological Grading

The definitions of the G categories apply to all digestive system tumours. These are:

G – Histopathological Grading
GX   Grade of differentiation cannot be assessed
G1   Well differentiated
G2   Moderately differentiated
G3   Poorly differentiated
G4   Undifferentiated

G4   Undifferentiated

R Classification

The absence or presence of residual tumour after treatment may be described by the symbol R. The definitions of the R classification apply to all digestive system tumours. These are:

- RX   Presence of residual tumour cannot be assessed
- R0   No residual tumour
- R1   Microscopic residual tumour
- R2   Macroscopic residual tumour

Oesophagus
(ICD-O C15)

Rules for Classification

The classification applies only to carcinomas. There should be histological confirmation of the disease and division of cases by histological type.

The following are the procedures for assessing T, N, and M categories.

T categories	Physical examination, imaging, endoscopy (including bronchoscopy), and/or surgical exploration
N categories	Physical examination, imaging, and/or surgical exploration
M categories	Physical examination, imaging, and/or surgical exploration

Anatomical Subsites

1. Cervical oesophagus (C15.0): This commences at the lower border of the cricoid cartilage and ends at the thoracic inlet (suprasternal notch), approximately 18 cm from the upper incisor teeth.
2. Intrathoracic oesophagus
    (i) The upper thoracic portion (C15.3) extending from the thoracic inlet to the level of the tracheal bifurcation, approximately 24 cm from the upper incisor teeth
    (ii) The mid-thoracic portion (C15.4) is the proximal half of the oesophagus between the tracheal bifurcation and the oesophagogastric junction. The lower

level is approximately 32 cm from the upper incisor teeth.

(iii) The lower thoracic portion (C15.5), approximately 8 cm in length (includes abdominal oesophagus), is the distal half of the oesophagus between the tracheal bifurcation and the oesophagogastric junction. The lower level is approximately 40 cm from the upper incisor teeth.

Regional Lymph Nodes

The regional lymph nodes are, for the cervical oesophagus, the cervical nodes including supraclavicular nodes, and, for the intrathoracic oesophagus, the mediastinal and perigastric nodes, excluding the coeliac nodes.

TNM Clinical Classification

T – Primary Tumour

TX Primary tumour cannot be assessed
T0 No evidence of primary tumour
Tis Carcinoma in situ

T1 Tumour invades lamina propria or submucosa
T2 Tumour invades muscularis propria
T3 Tumour invades adventitia
T4 Tumour invades adjacent structures

N – Regional Lymph Nodes

NX Regional lymph nodes cannot be assessed
N0 No regional lymph node metastasis
N1 Regional lymph node metastasis

M – Distant Metastasis

MX   Distant metastasis cannot be assessed

M0   No distant metastasis

M1   Distant metastasis

For tumours of lower thoracic oesophagus

M1a   Metastasis in coeliac lymph nodes

M1b   Other distant metastasis

For tumours of upper thoracic oesophagus

M1a   Metastasis in cervical lymph nodes

M1b   Other distant metastasis

For tumours of mid-thoracic oesphagus

M1a   Not applicable

M1b   Non-regional lymph node or other distant metastasis

pTNM Pathological Classification

The pT, pN, and pM categories correspond to the T, N, and M categories.

pN0 Histological examination of a mediastinal lymphadenectomy specimen will ordinarily include 6 or more lymph nodes.

G Histopathological Grading

See definitions on page 52.

Stage Grouping

Stage 0	Tis	N0	M0
Stage I	T1	N0	M0
Stage IIA	T2	N0	M0
	T3	N0	M0
Stage IIB	T1	N1	M0
	T2	N1	M0
Stage III	T3	N1	M0
	T4	Any N	M0
Stage IV	Any T	Any N	M1
Stage IVA	Any T	Any N	M1a
Stage IVB	Any T	Any N	M1b

Summary

Oesophagus	
T1	Lamina propria, submucosa
T2	Muscularis propria
T3	Adventitia
T4	Adjacent structures
N1	Regional
M1	Distant metastasis
	Tumour of lower thoracic oesophagus
M1a	Coeliac nodes
M1b	Other distant metastasis
	Tumour of upper thoracic oesophagus
M1a	Cervical nodes
M1b	Other distant metastasis
	Tumour of mid-thoracic oesophagus
M1b	Distant metastasis including non-regional lymph nodes

Stomach
(ICD-O C16)

Rules for Classification

The classification applies only to carcinomas. There should be histological confirmation of the disease.

The following are the procedures for assessing T, N, and M categories.

T categories	Physical examination, imaging, endoscopy, and/or surgical exploration
N categories	Physical examination, imaging, and/or surgical exploration
M categories	Physical examination, imaging, and/or surgical exploration

Anatomical Subsites

1. Cardia (C16.0)
2. Fundus (C16.1)
3. Corpus (C16.2)
4. Antrum (C16.3) and pylorus (C16.4)

Regional Lymph Nodes

The regional lymph nodes are the perigastric nodes along the lesser and greater curvatures, the nodes along the left gastric, common hepatic, splenic, and coeliac arteries, and the hepato-duodenal nodes.

Involvement of other intra-abdominal lymph nodes such as retropancreatic, mesenteric, and para-aortic is classified as distant metastasis.

TNM Clinical Classification

T – Primary Tumour

TX   Primary tumour cannot be assessed

T0   No evidence of primary tumour

Tis   Carcinoma in situ: intraepithelial tumour without invasion of the lamina propria

T1   Tumour invades lamina propria or submucosa

T2   Tumour invades muscularis propria or subserosa[1]

T3   Tumour penetrates serosa (visceral peritoneum) without invasion of adjacent structures[1, 2, 3]

T4   Tumour invades adjacent structures[1, 2, 3]

Notes: 1. A tumour may penetrate muscularis propria with extension into the gastro-colic or gastrohepatic ligaments or the greater and lesser omentum without perforation of the visceral peritoneum covering these structures. In this case, the tumour is classified as T2. If there is perforation of the visceral peritoneum covering the gastric ligaments or omenta, the tumour is classified as T3.
2. The adjacent structures of the stomach are the spleen, transverse colon, liver, diaphragm, pancreas, abdominal wall, adrenal gland, kidney, small intestine, and retroperitoneum.
3. Intramural extension to the duodenum or oesophagus is classified by the depth of greatest invasion in any of these sites including stomach.

N – Regional Lymph Nodes

NX   Regional lymph nodes cannot be assessed

N0   No regional lymph node metastasis

N1   Metastasis in 1 to 6 regional lymph nodes

N2   Metastasis in 7 to 15 regional lymph nodes

N3   Metastasis in more than 15 regional lymph nodes

M – Distant Metastasis

MX   Distant metastasis cannot be assessed
M0   No distant metastasis
M1   Distant metastasis

pTNM Pathological Classification

The pT, pN, and pM categories correspond to the T, N, and M categories.

pN0 Histological examination of a regional lymphadenectomy specimen will ordinarily include 15 or more lymph nodes.

G Histopathological Grading

See definitions on page 52.

Stage Grouping

Stage 0	Tis	N0	M0
Stage IA	T1	N0	M0
Stage IB	T1	N1	M0
	T2	N0	M0
Stage II	T1	N2	M0
	T2	N1	M0
	T3	N0	M0
Stage IIIA	T2	N2	M0
	T3	N1	M0
	T4	N0	M0
Stage IIIB	T3	N2	M0
Stage IV	T4	N1, N2, N3	M0
	T1, T2, T3	N3	M0
	Any T	Any N	M1

Summary

Stomach	
T1	Lamina propria, submucosa
T2	Muscularis propria, subserosa
T3	Penetrates serosa
T4	Adjacent structures
N1	1 to 6 nodes
N2	7 to 15 nodes
N3	>15 nodes

Small Intestine
(ICD-O C17)

Rules for Classification

The classification applies only to carcinomas. There should be histological confirmation of the disease.

The following are the procedures for assessing T, N, and M categories.

T categories	Physical examination, imaging, endoscopy, and/or surgical exploration
N categories	Physical examination, imaging, and/or surgical exploration
M categories	Physical examination, imaging, and/or surgical exploration

Anatomical Subsites

1. Duodenum (C17.0)
2. Jejunum (C17.1)
3. Ileum (C17.2) (excludes ileocecal valve C18.0)

Note: This classification does not apply to carcinomas of the ampulla of Vater (see page 84).

Regional Lymph Nodes

The regional lymph nodes for the duodenum are the pancreaticoduodenal, pyloric, hepatic (pericholedochal, cystic, hilar), and superior mesenteric nodes.

The regional lymph nodes for the ileum and jejunum are the mesenteric nodes, including the superior mesenteric nodes, and, for the terminal ileum only, the ileocolic nodes including the posterior cecal nodes.

TNM Clinical Classification

T – Primary Tumour

TX   Primary tumour cannot be assessed
T0   No evidence of primary tumour
Tis   Carcinoma in situ

T1   Tumour invades lamina propria or submucosa
T2   Tumour invades muscularis propria
T3   Tumour invades through muscularis propria into sub-serosa or into non-peritonealized perimuscular tissue (mesentery or retroperitoneum*) with extension 2 cm or less
T4   Tumour perforates visceral peritoneum or directly invades other organs or structures (includes other loops of small intestine, mesentery, or retroperitoneum more than 2 cm and abdominal wall by way of serosa; for duodenum only, invasion of pancreas)

Note: *The non-peritonealized perimuscular tissue is, for jejunum and ileum, part of the mesentery and, for duodenum in areas where serosa is lacking, part of the retroperitoneum.

N – Regional Lymph Nodes

NX   Regional lymph nodes cannot be assessed
N0   No regional lymph node metastasis
N1   Regional lymph node metastasis

M – Distant Metastasis

MX   Distant metastasis cannot be assessed
M0   No distant metastasis
M1   Distant metastasis

pTNM Pathological Classification

The pT, pN, and pM categories correspond to the T, N, and M categories.

pN0 Histological examination of a regional lymphadenectomy specimen will ordinarily include 6 or more lymph nodes.

G Histopathological Grading

See definitions on page 52.

Stage Grouping

Stage 0	Tis	N0	M0
Stage I	T1	N0	M0
	T2	N0	M0
Stage II	T3	N0	M0
	T4	N0	M0
Stage III	Any T	N1	M0
Stage IV	Any T	Any N	M1

Summary

Small Intestine	
T1	Lamina propria, submucosa
T2	Muscularis propria
T3	Subserosa, non-peritonealized perimuscular tissues (mesentery, retroperitoneum) ≤2 cm
T4	Visceral peritoneum, other organs/structures (including mesentery, retroperitoneum) >2 cm
N1	Regional

Colon and Rectum
(ICD-O C18-C20)

Rules for Classification

The classification applies only to carcinomas. There should be histological confirmation of the disease.

The following are the procedures for assessing T, N, and M categories.

T categories	Physical examination, imaging, endoscopy, and/or surgical exploration
N categories	Physical examination, imaging, and/or surgical exploration
M categories	Physical examination, imaging, and/or surgical exploration

Anatomical Subsites

Colon
1. Appendix (18.1)
2. Cecum (C18.0)
3. Ascending colon (C18.2)
4. Hepatic flexure (C18.3)
5. Transverse colon (C18.4)
6. Splenic flexure (C18.5)
7. Descending colon (C18.6)
8. Sigmoid colon (C18.7)

Rectum
1. Rectosigmoid junction (C19.9)
2. Rectum (C20.9)

Regional Lymph Nodes

The regional lymph nodes are the pericolic and perirectal and those located along the ileocolic, right colic, middle colic, left colic, inferior mesenteric, superior rectal (hacmorrhoidal), and internal iliac arteries.

TNM Clinical Classification

T – Primary Tumour

TX   Primary tumour cannot be assessed
T0   No evidence of primary tumour
Tis Carcinoma in situ: intraepithelial or invasion of lamina propria[1]

T1   Tumour invades submucosa
T2   Tumour invades muscularis propria
T3   Tumour invades through muscularis propria into subserosa or into non-peritonealized pericolic or perirectal tissues
T4   Tumour directly invades other organs or structures[2] and/or perforates visceral peritoneum

Notes: 1. Tis includes cancer cells confined within the glandular basement membrane (intraepithelial) or lamina propria (intramucosal) with no extension through muscularis mucosae into submucosa.
2. Direct invasion in T4 includes invasion of other segments of the colorectum by way of the serosa, e.g. invasion of sigmoid colon by a carcinoma of the cecum.

N – Regional Lymph Nodes

NX   Regional lymph nodes cannot be assessed
N0   No regional lymph node metastasis
N1   Metastasis in 1 to 3 regional lymph nodes
N2   Metastasis in 4 or more regional lymph nodes

Note: A tumour nodule greater than 3 mm in diameter in perirectal or pericolic adipose tissue without histological evidence of a residual lymph node in the nodule is classified as regional lymph node metastasis. However, a tumour nodule up to 3 mm in diameter is classified in the T category as discontinuous extension, i.e., T3.

M – Distant Metastasis

MX   Distant metastasis cannot be assessed
M0   No distant metastasis
M1   Distant metastasis

pTNM Pathological Classification

The pT, pN, and pM categories correspond to the T, N, and M categories.

pN0 Histological examination of a regional lymphadenectomy specimen will ordinarily include 12 or more lymph nodes.

G Histopathological Grading

See definitions on page 52.

Stage Grouping

TNM				*Dukes*
Stage 0	Tis	N0	M0	
Stage I	T1	N0	M0	*A*
	T2	N0	M0	
Stage II	T3	N0	M0	*B**
	T4	N0	M0	
Stage III	Any T	N1	M0	*C**
	Any T	N2	M0	
Stage IV	Any T	Any N	M1	

Note: *Dukes B is a composite of better (T3N0M0) and worse (T4N0M0) prognostic groups, as is Dukes C (anyTN1M0 and anyTN2M0)

Summary

Colon and Rectum	
T1	Submucosa
T2	Muscularis propria
T3	Subserosa, non-peritonealized pericolic/perirectal tissues
T4	Other organs or structures/visceral peritoneum
N1	<3 regional
N2	>3 regional

Anal Canal
(ICD-O C21.1, 2)

The anal canal extends from rectum to perianal skin (to the junction with hair-bearing skin). It is lined by the mucous membrane overlying the internal sphincter, including the transitional epithelium and dentate line. Tumours of anal margin (ICD-O C44.5) are classified with skin tumours (page 111).

Rules for Classification

The classification applies only to carcinomas. There should be histological confirmation of the disease.

The following are the procedures for assessing T, N, and M categories.

T categories	Physical examination, imaging, endoscopy, and/or surgical exploration
N categories	Physical examination, imaging, and/or surgical exploration
M categories	Physical examination, imaging, and/or surgical exploration

Regional Lymph Nodes

The regional lymph nodes are the perirectal, the internal iliac, and the inguinal lymph nodes.

TNM Clinical Classification

T – Primary Tumour

TX   Primary tumour cannot be assessed
T0   No evidence of primary tumour
Tis   Carcinoma in situ

T1   Tumour 2 cm or less in greatest dimension
T2   Tumour more than 2 cm but not more than 5 cm in greatest dimension
T3   Tumour more than 5 cm in greatest dimension
T4   Tumour of any size invades adjacent organ(s), e.g., vagina, urethra, bladder (involvement of sphincter muscle(s) *alone* is not classified as T4)

N – Regional Lymph Nodes

NX   Regional lymph nodes cannot be assessed
N0   No regional lymph node metastasis
N1   Metastasis in perirectal lymph node(s)
N2   Metastasis in unilateral internal iliac and/or inguinal lymph node(s)
N3   Metastasis in perirectal and inguinal lymph nodes and/or bilateral internal iliac and/or inguinal lymph nodes

M – Distant Metastasis

MX   Distant metastasis cannot be assessed
M0   No distant metastasis
M1   Distant metastasis

pTNM Pathological Classification

The pT, pN, and pM categories correspond to the T, N, and M categories.

pN0 Histological examination of a regional perirectal-pelvic lymphadenectomy specimen will ordinarily include 12 or more lymph nodes; histological examination of an inguinal lymphadenectomy specimen will ordinarily include 6 or more lymph nodes.

G Histopathological Grading

See definitions on page 52.

Stage Grouping

Stage 0	Tis	N0	M0
Stage I	T1	N0	M0
Stage II	T2	N0	M0
	T3	N0	M0
Stage IIIA	T1	N1	M0
	T2	N1	M0
	T3	N1	M0
	T4	N0	M0
Stage IIIB	T4	N1	M0
	Any T	N2, N3	M0
Stage IV	Any T	Any N	M1

Summary

Anal Canal	
T1	≤2 cm
T2	>2 to 5 cm
T3	>5 cm
T4	Adjacent organ(s)
N1	Perirectal
N2	Unilateral internal iliac/inguinal
N3	Perirectal and inguinal, bilateral internal iliac/inguinal

Liver
(ICD-O C22)

Rules for Classification

The classification applies only to primary hepatocellular and cholangio- (intrahepatic bile duct) carcinoma of the liver. There should be histological confirmation of the disease and division of cases by histological type.

The following are the procedures for assessing T, N, and M categories.

T categories	Physical examination, imaging, and/or surgical exploration
N categories	Physical examination, imaging, and/or surgical exploration
M categories	Physical examination, imaging, and/or surgical exploration

Note: Although the presence of cirrhosis is an important prognostic factor it does not affect the TNM classification, being an independent prognostic variable.

Anatomical Subsites

1. Liver (C22.0)
2. Intrahepatic bile duct (C22.1)

Regional Lymph Nodes

The regional lymph nodes are the hilar nodes (i.e., those in the hepatoduodenal ligament).

TNM Clinical Classification

T – Primary Tumour

TX   Primary tumour cannot be assessed

T0   No evidence of primary tumour

T1   Solitary tumour 2 cm or less in greatest dimension without vascular invasion

T2   Solitary tumour 2 cm or less in greatest dimension with vascular invasion; *or* multiple tumours limited to one lobe, none more than 2 cm in greatest dimension without vascular invasion; *or* solitary tumour more than 2 cm in greatest dimension without vascular invasion

T3   Solitary tumour more than 2 cm in greatest dimension with vascular invasion; *or* multiple tumours limited to one lobe, none more than 2 cm in greatest dimension with vascular invasion; *or* multiple tumours limited to one lobe, any more than 2 cm in greatest dimension with or without vascular invasion.

T4   Multiple tumours in more than one lobe; *or* tumour(s) involve(s) a major branch of the portal or hepatic vein(s); *or* tumour(s) with direct invasion of adjacent organs other than gallbladder; *or* tumour(s) with perforation of visceral peritoneum.

Note: For classification, the plane projecting between the bed of the gallbladder and the inferior vena cava divides the liver in two lobes.

N – Regional Lymph Nodes

NX   Regional lymph nodes cannot be assessed

N0   No regional lymph node metastasis

N1   Regional lymph node metastasis

M – Distant Metastasis

    MX   Distant metastasis cannot be assessed
    M0   No distant metastasis
    M1   Distant metastasis

pTNM Pathological Classification

The pT, pN, and pM categories correspond to the T, N, and M categories.

   pN0 Histological examination of a regional lymphadenectomy specimen will ordinarily include 3 or more lymph nodes.

G Histopathological Grading

See definitions on page 52.

Stage Grouping

Stage I	T1	N0	M0
Stage II	T2	N0	M0
Stage IIIA	T3	N0	M0
Stage IIIB	T1	N1	M0
	T2	N1	M0
	T3	N1	M0
Stage IVA	T4	Any N	M0
Stage IVB	Any T	Any N	M1

Summary

Liver	
T1	Solitary, ≤2 cm, without vascular invasion
T2	Solitary, ≤2 cm, with vascular invasion Multiple, one lobe, ≤2 cm, without vascular invasion Solitary, >2 cm, without vascular invasion
T3	Solitary, >2 cm, with vascular invasion Multiple, one lobe, ≤2 cm, with vascular invasion Multiple, one lobe, >2 cm, with or without vascular invasion
T4	Multiple, more than one lobe Invasion of major branch of portal or hepatic veins Invasion of adjacent organs other than gallbladder Perforation of visceral peritoneum
N1	Regional

Gallbladder
(ICD-O C23.9)

Rules for Classification

The classification applies only to carcinomas. There should be histological confirmation of the disease.

The following are the procedures for assessing T, N, and M categories.

T categories	Physical examination, imaging, and/or surgical exploration
N categories	Physical examination, imaging, and/or surgical exploration
M categories	Physical examination, imaging, and/or surgical exploration

Regional Lymph Nodes

The regional lymph nodes are the cystic duct node and the pericholedochal, hilar, peripancreatic (head only), periduodenal, periportal, coeliac, and superior mesenteric nodes.

TNM Clinical Classification

T – Primary Tumour

TX   Primary tumour cannot be assessed
T0   No evidence of primary tumour
Tis   Carcinoma in situ

T1   Tumour invades lamina propria or muscle layer
    T1a   Tumour invades lamina propria
    T1b   Tumour invades muscle layer
T2   Tumour invades perimuscular connective tissue, no extension beyond serosa or into liver
T3   Tumour perforates serosa (visceral peritoneum) or directly invades into one adjacent organ or both (extension 2 cm or less into liver)
T4   Tumour extends more than 2 cm into liver and/or into two or more adjacent organs (stomach, duodenum, colon, pancreas, omentum, extrahepatic bile ducts, any involvement of liver)

N – Regional Lymph Nodes

NX   Regional lymph nodes cannot be assessed
N0   No regional lymph node metastasis
N1   Metastasis in cystic duct, pericholedochal, and/or hilar lymph nodes (i.e., in the hepatoduodenal ligament)
N2   Metastasis in peripancreatic (head only), periduodenal, periportal, coeliac, and/or superior mesenteric lymph nodes

M – Distant Metastasis

MX   Distant metastasis cannot be assessed
M0   No distant metastasis
M1   Distant metastasis

pTNM Pathological Classification

The pT, pN, and pM categories correspond to the T, N, and M categories.

pN0 Histological examination of a regional lymphadenectomy specimen will ordinarily include 3 or more lymph nodes.

G Histopathological Grading

See definitions on page 52.

Stage Grouping

Stage 0	Tis	N0	M0
Stage I	T1	N0	M0
Stage II	T2	N0	M0
Stage III	T1	N1	M0
	T2	N1	M0
	T3	N0, N1	M0
Stage IVA	T4	N0, N1	M0
Stage IVB	Any T	N2	M0
	Any T	Any N	M1

Summary

Gallbladder	
T1	Gallbladder wall
T1a	Lamina propria
T1b	Muscle
T2	Perimuscular connective tissue
T3	Serosa and/or one organ, liver ≤2 cm
T4	Two or more organs, or liver >2 cm
N1	Hepatoduodenal ligament
N2	Other regional

Extrahepatic Bile Ducts
(ICD-O C24.0)

Rules for Classification

The classification applies to carcinomas of extrahepatic bile ducts and those of choledochal cysts. There should be histological confirmation of the disease.

The following are the procedures for assessing T, N, and M categories.

T categories	Physical examination, imaging, and/or surgical exploration
N categories	Physical examination, imaging, and/or surgical exploration
M categories	Physical examination, imaging, and/or surgical exploration

Regional Lymph Nodes

The regional lymph nodes are the cystic duct, pericholedochal, hilar, peripancreatic (head only), periduodenal, periportal, coeliac, and superior mesenteric nodes.

TNM Clinical Classification

T – Primary Tumour

TX Primary tumour cannot be assessed
T0 No evidence of primary tumour
Tis Carcinoma in situ

T1   Tumour invades subepithelial connective tissue or fibromuscular layer

    T1a   Tumour invades subepithelial connective tissue

    T1b   Tumour invades fibromuscular layer

T2   Tumour invades perifibromuscular connective tissue

T3   Tumour invades adjacent structures: liver, pancreas, duodenum, gallbladder, colon, stomach

N – Regional Lymph Nodes

NX   Regional lymph nodes cannot be assessed

N0   No regional lymph node metastasis

N1   Metastasis in cystic duct, pericholedochal, and/or hilar lymph nodes (i.e., in the hepatoduodenal ligament)

N2   Metastasis in peripancreatic (head only), periduodenal, periportal, coeliac, superior mesenteric, posterior peripancreatico-duodenal lymph nodes

M – Distant Metastasis

MX   Distant metastasis cannot be assessed

M0   No distant metastasis

M1   Distant metastasis

pTNM Pathological Classification

The pT, pN, and pM categories correspond to the T, N, and M categories.

pN0 Histological examination of a regional lymphadenectomy specimen will ordinarily include 3 or more lymph nodes.

G Histopathological Grading

See definitions on page 52.

Stage Grouping

Stage 0	Tis	N0	M0
Stage I	T1	N0	M0
Stage II	T2	N0	M0
Stage III	T1	N1, N2	M0
	T2	N1, N2	M0
Stage IVA	T3	Any N	M0
Stage IVB	Any T	Any N	M1

Summary

Extrahepatic Bile Ducts	
T1	Ductal wall
T1a	Subepithclial connective tissue
T1b	Fibromuscular layer
T2	Perifibromuscular connective tissue
T3	Adjacent structures
N1	Hepatoduodenal ligament
N2	Other regional

Ampulla of Vater
(ICD-O C24.1)

Rules for Classification

The classification applies only to carcinomas. There should be histological confirmation of the disease.

The following are the procedures for assessing T, N, and M categories.

T categories	Physical examination, imaging, and/or surgical exploration
N categories	Physical examination, imaging, and/or surgical exploration
M categories	Physical examination, imaging, and/or surgical exploration

Regional Lymph Nodes

The regional lymph nodes are:

Superior	Superior to head and body of pancreas
Inferior	Inferior to head and body of pancreas
Anterior	Anterior pancreaticoduodenal, pyloric, and proximal mesenteric
Posterior	Posterior pancreaticoduodenal, common bile duct, and proximal mesenteric

Note: The splenic lymph nodes and those of the tail of the pancreas are *not* regional; metastases to these lymph nodes are coded M1.

TNM Clinical Classification

T – Primary Tumour

TX Primary tumour cannot be assessed
T0 No evidence of primary tumour
Tis Carcinoma in situ

T1 Tumour limited to ampulla of Vater or sphincter of Oddi
T2 Tumour invades duodenal wall
T3 Tumour invades 2 cm or less into pancreas
T4 Tumour invades more than 2 cm into pancreas and/or into other adjacent organs

N – Regional Lymph Nodes

NX Regional lymph nodes cannot be assessed
N0 No regional lymph node metastasis
N1 Regional lymph node metastasis

M – Distant Metastasis

MX Distant metastasis cannot be assessed
M0 No distant metastasis
M1 Distant metastasis

pTNM Pathological Classification

The pT, pN, and pM categories correspond to the T, N, and M categories.

pN0 Histological examination of a regional lymphadenectomy specimen will ordinarily include 10 or more lymph nodes.

G Histopathological Grading

See definitions on page 52.

Stage Grouping

Stage 0	Tis	N0	M0
Stage I	T1	N0	M0
Stage II	T2	N0	M0
	T3	N0	M0
Stage III	T1	N1	M0
	T2	N1	M0
	T3	N1	M0
Stage IV	T4	Any N	M0
	Any T	Any N	M1

Summary

Ampulla of Vater	
T1	Ampulla or sphincter of Oddi
T2	Duodenal wall
T3	Pancreas ≤2 cm
T4	Pancreas >2 cm, other organs
N1	Regional

Pancreas
(ICD-O C25.0-2, 8)

Rules for Classification

The classification applies only to carcinomas of the exocrine pancreas. There should be histological or cytological confirmation of the disease.

The following are the procedures for assessing T, N, and M categories.

T categories	Physical examination, imaging, and/or surgical exploration
N categories	Physical examination, imaging, and/or surgical exploration
M categories	Physical examination, imaging, and/or surgical exploration

Anatomical Subsites

1. Head of pancreas[1] (C25.0)
2. Body of pancreas[2] (C25.1)
3. Tail of pancreas[3] (C25.2)
4. Entire pancreas (C25.8)

Notes: 1. Tumours of the head of the pancreas are those arising to the right of the left border of the superior mesenteric vein. The uncinate process is considered as part of the head.
2. Tumours of the body are those arising between the left border of the superior mesenteric vein and left border of the aorta.
3. Tumours of the tail are those arising between the left border of the aorta and the hilum of the spleen.

Regional Lymph Nodes

The regional lymph nodes are the peripancreatic nodes, which may be subdivided as follows:

Superior	Superior to head and body
Inferior	Inferior to head and body
Anterior	Anterior pancreaticoduodenal, pyloric (for tumours of head only), and proximal mesenteric
Posterior	Posterior pancreaticoduodenal, common bile duct, and proximal mesenteric
Splenic	Hilum of spleen and tail of pancreas (for tumours of body and tail only)
Coeliac	(for tumours of head only)

TNM Clinical Classification

T – Primary Tumour

TX   Primary tumour cannot be assessed

T0   No evidence of primary tumour

Tis   Carcinoma in situ

T1   Tumour limited to the pancreas, 2 cm or less in greatest dimension

T2   Tumour limited to the pancreas, more than 2 cm in greatest dimension

T3   Tumour extends directly into any of the following: duodenum, bile duct, peripancreatic tissues[1]

T4   Tumour extends directly into any of the following: stomach, spleen, colon, adjacent large vessels[2]

Note: 1. Peripancreatic tissues include the surrounding retroperitoneal fat (retroperitoneal soft tissue or retroperitoneal space), including mesentery (mesenteric fat), mesocolon, greater and lesser omentum, and peritoneum. Direct invasion to bile ducts and duodenum includes involvement of ampulla of Vater.
2. Adjacent large vessels are the portal vein, coeliac artery, and superior mesenteric and common hepatic arteries and veins (not splenic vessels).

N – Regional Lymph Nodes

NX   Regional lymph nodes cannot be assessed
N0   No regional lymph node metastasis
N1   Regional lymph node metastasis
    N1a   Metastasis in a single regional lymph node
    N1b   Metastasis in multiple regional lymph nodes

M – Distant Metastasis

MX   Distant metastasis cannot be assessed
M0   No distant metastasis
M1   Distant metastasis

pTNM Pathological Classification

The pT, pN, and pM categories correspond to the T, N, and M categories.

pN0 Histological examination of a regional lymphadenectomy specimen will ordinarily include 10 or more lymph nodes.

G Histopathological Grading

See definitions on page 52.

Stage Grouping

Stage 0	Tis	N0	M0
Stage I	T1	N0	M0
	T2	N0	M0
Stage II	T3	N0	M0
Stage III	T1	N1	M0
	T2	N1	M0
	T3	N1	M0
Stage IVA	T4	Any N	M0
Stage IVB	Any T	Any N	M1

Summary

Pancreas	
T1	Limited to the pancreas ≤2 cm
T2	Limited to the pancreas >2 cm
T3	Duodenum, bile duct, peripancreatic tissues
T4	Stomach, spleen, colon, large vessels
N1	Regional
N1a	Single node
N1b	Multiple nodes

LUNG AND PLEURAL TUMOURS

Introductory Notes

The classifications apply to carcinomas of the lung and malignant mesothelioma of pleura.

Each site is described under the following headings:

- Rules for classification with the procedures for assessing T, N, and M categories; additional methods may be used when they enhance the accuracy of appraisal before treatment
- Anatomical subsites where appropriate
- Definition of the regional lymph nodes
- TNM Clinical classification
- TNM Pathological classification
- G Histopathological grading where applicable
- Stage grouping
- Summary

Regional Lymph Nodes

Six lymph nodes ordinarily are included in a hilar or mediastinal lymphadenectomy specimen. The designation pN0 is usually based on this figure.

Distant Metastasis

The categories M1 and pM1 may be further specified according to the following notation:

Pulmonary	PUL	Bone marrow	MAR
Osseous	OSS	Pleura	PLE
Hepatic	HEP	Peritoneum	PER
Brain	BRA	Adrenals	ADR
Lymph nodes	LYM	Skin	SKI
Others	OTH		

R Classification

The absence or presence of residual tumour after treatment may be described by the symbol R. The definitions of the R classification are:

RX Presence of residual tumour cannot be assessed
R0 No residual tumour
R1 Microscopic residual tumour
R2 Macroscopic residual tumour

Lung
(ICD-O C34)

Rules for Classification

The classification applies only to carcinomas. There should be histological confirmation of the disease and division of cases by histological type.

The following are the procedures for assessing T, N, and M categories:

T categories	Physical examination, imaging, endoscopy, and/or surgical exploration
N categories	Physical examination, imaging, endoscopy, and/or surgical exploration
M categories	Physical examination, imaging, and/or surgical exploration

Anatomical Subsites

1. Main bronchus (C34.0)
2. Upper lobe (C34.1)
3. Middle lobe (C34.2)
4. Lower lobe (C34.3)

Regional Lymph Nodes

The regional lymph nodes are the intrathoracic, scalene, and supraclavicular nodes.

TNM Clinical Classification

T – Primary Tumour

TX   Primary tumour cannot be assessed, *or* tumour proven by the pres-
      ence of malignant cells in sputum or bronchial washings but not
      visualized by imaging or bronchoscopy

T0   No evidence of primary tumour

Tis   Carcinoma in situ

T1   Tumour 3 cm or less in greatest dimension, sur-
      rounded by lung or visceral pleura, without broncho-
      scopic evidence of invasion more proximal than the
      lobar bronchus (i.e., not in the main bronchus)[1]

T2   Tumour with *any* of the following features of size or
      extent:
      • More than 3 cm in greatest dimension
      • Involves main bronchus, 2 cm or more distal to the
        carina
      • Invades visceral pleura
      • Associated with atelectasis or obstructive pneu-
        monitis that extends to the hilar region but does not
        involve the entire lung

T3   Tumour of any size that directly invades any of the
      following: chest wall (including superior sulcus
      tumours), diaphragm, mediastinal pleura, parietal
      pericardium; *or* tumour in the main bronchus less than
      2 cm distal to the carina[1] but without involvement of
      the carina; *or* associated atelectasis or obstructive
      pneumonitis of the entire lung

T4   Tumour of any size that invades any of the following:
      mediastinum, heart, great vessels, trachea, oesopha-
      gus, vertebral body, carina; separate tumour nodule(s)
      in the same lobe; tumour with malignant pleural effu-
      sion[2]

Notes: 1. The uncommon superficial spreading tumour of any size with its invasive
component limited to the bronchial wall, which may extend proximal to the
main bronchus, is also classified as T1.

2. Most pleural effusions with lung cancer are due to tumour. In a few
patients, however, multiple cytopathological examinations of pleural fluid
are negative for tumour, and the fluid is non-bloody and is not an exudate.
Where these elements and clinical judgment dictate that the effusion is not
related to the tumour, the effusion should be excluded as a staging element
and the patient should be classified as T1, T2, or T3.

N – Regional Lymph Nodes

NX   Regional lymph nodes cannot be assessed

N0   No regional lymph node metastasis

N1   Metastasis in ipsilateral peribronchial and/or ipsilateral hilar lymph nodes and intrapulmonary nodes,
including involvement by direct extension

N2   Metastasis in ipsilateral mediastinal and/or subcarinal
lymph node(s)

N3   Metastasis in contralateral mediastinal, contralateral
hilar, ipsilateral or contralateral scalene, or supraclavicular lymph node(s)

M – Distant Metastasis

MX   Distant metastasis cannot be assessed

M0   No distant metastasis

M1   Distant metastasis, includes separate tumour nodule(s)
in a different lobe (ipsilateral or contralateral)

pTNM Pathological Classification

The pT, pN, and pM categories correspond to the T, N, and M
categories.

pN0 Histological examination of hilar and mediastinal
lymphadenectomy specimen(s) will ordinarily include 6 or
more lymph nodes.

G Histopathological Grading

GX   Grade of differentiation cannot be assessed
G1   Well differentiated
G2   Moderately differentiated
G3   Poorly differentiated
G4   Undifferentiated

Stage Grouping

Occult carcinoma	TX	N0	M0
Stage 0	Tis	N0	M0
Stage IA	T1	N0	M0
Stage IB	T2	N0	M0
Stage IIA	T1	N1	M0
Stage IIB	T2	N1	M0
	T3	N0	M0
Stage IIIA	T1	N2	M0
	T2	N2	M0
	T3	N1, N2	M0
Stage IIIB	Any T	N3	M0
	T4	Any N	M0
Stage IV	Any T	Any N	M1

Summary

Lung	
TX	Positive cytology
T1	≤3 cm
T2	>3 cm, main bronchus ≥2 cm from carina, invades visceral pleura, partial atelectasis
T3	Chest wall, diaphragm, pericardium, mediastinal pleura, main bronchus <2 cm from carina, total atelectasis
T4	Mediastinum, heart, great vessels, carina, trachea, oesophagus, vertebra; separate nodules in same lobe, malignant effusion
N1	Ipsilateral peribronchial, ipsilateral hilar
N2	Ipsilateral mediastinal, subcarinal
N3	Contralateral mediastinal or hilar, scalene or supraclavicular
M1	Includes separate nodule in different lobe

Pleural Mesothelioma
(ICD-O C38.4)

Rules for Classification

The classification applies only to malignant mesothelioma of the pleura. There should be histological confirmation of the disease.

The following are the procedures for assessing T, N, and M categories:

T categories	Physical examination, imaging, endoscopy, and/or surgical exploration
N categories	Physical examination, imaging, endoscopy, and/or surgical exploration
M categories	Physical examination, imaging, and/or surgical exploration

Regional Lymph Nodes

The regional lymph nodes are the intrathoracic, scalene, and supraclavicular nodes.

TNM Clinical Classification

T – Primary Tumour

TX   Primary tumour cannot be assessed
T0   No evidence of primary tumour

T1 Tumour limited to ipsilateral parietal and/or visceral pleura

T2 Tumour invades any of the following: ipsilateral lung, endothoracic fascia, diaphragm, pericardium

T3 Tumour invades any of the following: ipsilateral chest wall muscle, ribs, mediastinal organs or tissues

T4 Tumour directly extends to any of the following: contralateral pleura, contralateral lung, peritoneum, intra-abdominal organs, cervical tissues

N – Regional Lymph Nodes

NX Regional lymph nodes cannot be assessed

N0 No regional lymph node metastasis

N1 Metastasis in ipsilateral peribronchial and/or ipsilateral hilar lymph nodes, including involvement by direct extension

N2 Metastasis in ipsilateral mediastinal and/or subcarinal lymph node(s)

N3 Metastasis in contralateral mediastinal, contralateral hilar, ipsilateral or contralateral scalene, or supraclavicular lymph node(s)

M – Distant Metastasis

MX Distant metastasis cannot be assessed

M0 No distant metastasis

M1 Distant metastasis

pTNM Pathological Classification

The pT, pN, and pM categories correspond to the T, N, and M categories.

Stage Grouping

Stage I	T1	N0	M0
	T2	N0	M0
Stage II	T1	N1	M0
	T2	N1	M0
Stage III	T1	N2	M0
	T2	N2	M0
	T3	N0, N1, N2	M0
Stage IV	Any T	N3	M0
	T4	Any N	M0
	Any T	Any N	M1

Summary

Pleural Mesothelioma	
T1	Ipsilateral pleura
T2	Ipsilateral lung, endothoracic fascia, diaphragm, pericardium
T3	Ipsilateral chest wall muscle, ribs, mediastinal organs or tissues
T4	Direct extension to contralateral pleura, lung, peritoneum, intra-abdominal organs, cervical tissue
N1	Ipsilateral peribronchial, ipsilateral hilar
N2	Ipsilateral mediastinal, subcarinal
N3	Contralateral mediastinal or hilar, scalene, or supraclavicular

TUMOURS OF BONE AND SOFT TISSUES

Introductory Notes

The following sites are included:
- Bone
- Soft tissue

Each site is described under the following headings:

- Rules for classification with the procedures for assessing T, N, and M categories; additional methods may be used when they enhance the accuracy of appraisal before treatment
- Anatomical sites where appropriate
- Definition of the regional lymph nodes
- TNM Clinical classification
- pTNM Pathological classification
- G Histopathological grading
- Stage grouping
- Summary

Distant Metastasis

The categories M1 and pM1 may be further specified according to the following notation:

Pulmonary	PUL	Bone marrow	MAR
Osseous	OSS	Pleura	PLE
Hepatic	HEP	Peritoneum	PER
Brain	BRA	Adrenals	ADR
Lymph nodes	LYM	Skin	SKI
Others	OTH		

R Classification

The absence or presence of residual tumour after treatment may be described by the symbol R. The definitions of the R classification are:

RX   Presence of residual tumour cannot be assessed
R0   No residual tumour
R1   Microscopic residual tumour
R2   Macroscopic residual tumour

Bone
(ICD-O C40, 41)

Rules for Classification

The classification applies to all primary malignant bone tumours except malignant lymphomas, multiple myeloma, surface/juxtacortical osteosarcoma, and juxtacortical chondrosarcoma. There should be histological confirmation of the disease and division of cases by histological type and grade.

The following are the procedures for assessing T, N, and M categories:

T categories	Physical examination and imaging
N categories	Physical examination and imaging
M categories	Physical examination and imaging

Regional Lymph Nodes

The regional lymph nodes are those appropriate to the site of the primary tumour.

TNM Clinical Classification

T – Primary Tumour
TX   Primary tumour cannot be assessed
T0   No evidence of primary tumour

T1   Tumour confined within the cortex
T2   Tumour invades beyond the cortex

N – Regional Lymph Nodes

NX   Regional lymph nodes cannot be assessed
N0   No regional lymph node metastasis
N1   Regional lymph node metastasis

M – Distant Metastasis

MX   Distant metastasis cannot be assessed
M0   No distant metastasis
M1   Distant metastasis

pTNM Pathological Classification

The pT, pN, and pM categories correspond to the T, N, and M categories.

G Histopathological Grading

GX   Grade of differentiation cannot be assessed
G1   Well differentiated
G2   Moderately differentiated
G3   Poorly differentiated
G4   Undifferentiated

Note: Ewing sarcoma is classified as G4.

Stage Grouping

Stage IA	G1, 2	T1	N0	M0
Stage IB	G1, 2	T2	N0	M0
Stage IIA	G3, 4	T1	N0	M0
Stage IIB	G3, 4	T2	N0	M0
Stage III	Not defined			
Stage IVA	Any G	Any T	N1	M0
Stage IVB	Any G	Any T	Any N	M1

Summary

Bone	
T1	Within cortex
T2	Beyond cortex
N1	Regional
G1	Well differentiated
G2	Moderately differentiated
G3	Poorly differentiated
G4	Undifferentiated

Soft Tissues
(ICD-O C38.1, 2, C47-49)

Rules for Classification

There should be histological confirmation of the disease and division of cases by histological type and grade.

The following are the procedures for assessing T, N, and M categories:

T categories	Physical examination and imaging
N categories	Physical examination and imaging
M categories	Physical examination and imaging

Anatomical Sites

1. Connective, subcutaneous, and other soft tissues, peripheral nerves (C47, C49)
2. Retroperitoneum (C48)
3. Mediastinum (C38.1, 2)

Histological Types of Tumour

The following histological types of malignant tumour are included, the appropriate ICD-O morphology rubrics being indicated:

Alveolar soft part sarcoma	9581/3
Angiosarcoma	9120/3
Epithelioid sarcoma	8804/3
Extraskeletal chondrosarcoma	9220/3
Extraskeletal osteosarcoma	9180/3

Fibrosarcoma	8810/3
Leiomyosarcoma	8890/3
Liposarcoma	8850/3
Malignant fibrous histiocytoma	8830/3
Malignant hemangiopericytoma	9150/3
Malignant mesenchymoma	8990/3
Malignant schwannoma	9560/3
Rhabdomyosarcoma	8900/3
Synovial sarcoma	9040/3
Sarcoma NOS (not otherwise specified)	8800/3

The following histological types of tumour are not included: Kaposi sarcoma, dermatofibrosarcoma (protuberans), fibrosarcoma grade I (desmoid tumour), and sarcoma arising from the dura mater, brain, parenchymatous organs, or hollow viscera.

Regional Lymph Nodes

The regional lymph nodes are those appropriate to the site of the primary tumour.

TNM Clinical Classification

T – Primary Tumour

TX   Primary tumour cannot be assessed
T0   No evidence of primary tumour

T1   Tumour 5 cm or less in greatest dimension
    T1a   Superficial tumour*
    T1b   Deep tumour*

T2   Tumour more than 5 cm in greatest dimension
     T2a   Superficial tumour*
     T2b   Deep tumour*

Note: *Superficial tumour is located exclusively above the superficial fascia without invasion of the fascia; deep tumour is located either exclusively beneath the superficial fascia or superficial to the fascia with invasion of or through the fascia. Retroperitoneal, mediastinal, and pelvic sarcomas are classified as deep tumours.

N – Regional Lymph Nodes

NX   Regional lymph nodes cannot be assessed
N0   No regional lymph node metastasis
N1   Regional lymph node metastasis

M – Distant Metastasis

MX   Distant metastasis cannot be assessed
M0   No distant metastasis
M1   Distant metastasis

pTNM Pathological Classification

The pT, pN, and pM categories correspond to the T, N, and M categories.

G Histopathological Grading

GX   Grade of differentiation cannot be assessed
G1   Well differentiated
G2   Moderately differentiated
G3   Poorly differentiated
G4   Undifferentiated

Note: After the histological type has been determined, the tumour should be graded according to the accepted criteria including cellularity, cellular pleomorphism, mitotic activity, and necrosis. The amount of intercellular substance such as collagen or mucoid material should be considered as a favourable factor in assessing the grade.

Stage Grouping

Stage IA	G1, 2	T1a	N0	M0
	G1, 2	T1b	N0	M0
Stage IB	G1, 2	T2a	N0	M0
Stage IIA	G1, 2	T2b	N0	M0
Stage IIB	G3, 4	T1a	N0	M0
	G3, 4	T1b	N0	M0
Stage IIC	G3, 4	T2a	N0	M0
Stage III	G3, 4	T2b	N0	M0
Stage IV	Any G	Any T	N1	M0
	Any G	Any T	Any N	M1

Summary

Soft Tissue Sarcoma	

T1
  T1a
  T1b
	≤5 cm
	  Superficial
	  Deep

T2
  T2a
  T2b
	>5 cm
	  Superficial
	  Deep

N1	Regional
G1	Well differentiated
G2	Moderately differentiated
G3	Poorly differentiated
G4	Undifferentiated

SKIN TUMOURS

Introductory Notes

The classifications apply to carcinomas of the skin, excluding eyelid (see page 198), vulva (see page 134), and penis (see page 167) and to malignant melanomas of the skin including eyelid.

Anatomical Sites

The following sites are identified by ICD-O topography rubrics:

- Lip (excluding vermilion surface) (C44.0)
- Eyelid (C44.1)
- External ear (C44.2)
- Other and unspecified parts of face (C44.3)
- Scalp and neck (C44.4)
- Trunk including anal margin and perianal skin (C44.5)
- Upper limb and shoulder (C44.6)
- Lower limb and hip (C44.7)
- Vulva (C51.0)
- Penis (C60.9)
- Scrotum (C63.2)

Each tumour type is described under the following headings:

- Rules for classification with the procedures for assessing T, N, and M categories
- Regional lymph nodes
- TNM Clinical classification
- pTNM Pathological classification
- G Histopathological grading where applicable
- Stage grouping
- Summary

Regional Lymph Nodes

The regional lymph nodes are those appropriate to the site of the primary tumour.

Unilateral Tumours
- **Head, neck:** Ipsilateral preauricular, submandibular, cervical, and supraclavicular lymph nodes
- **Thorax:** Ipsilateral axillary lymph nodes
- **Upper limb:** Ipsilateral epitrochlear and axillary lymph nodes
- **Abdomen, loins, and buttocks**: Ipsilateral inguinal lymph nodes
- **Lower limb:** Ipsilateral popliteal and inguinal lymph nodes
- **Anal margin and perianal skin:** Ipsilateral inguinal lymph nodes

Tumours in the Boundary Zones Between the Above
The lymph nodes pertaining to the regions on both sides of the boundary zone are considered to be the regional lymph nodes.

The following 4-cm-wide bands are considered as boundary zones:

Between	Along
Right/left	Midline
Head and neck/thorax	Clavicula–acromion–upper shoulder blade edge
Thorax/upper limb	Shoulder–axilla–shoulder
Thorax/abdomen, loins, and buttocks	*Front:* middle between navel and costal arch *Back:* lower border of thoracic vertebrae (midtransverse axis)
Abdomen, loins, and buttock/lower limb	Groin–trochanter–gluteal sulcus

Any metastasis to other than the listed regional lymph nodes is considered as M1.

Distant Metastasis

The categories M1 and pM1 may be further specified according to the following notation:

Pulmonary	PUL	Bone marrow	MAR
Osseous	OSS	Pleura	PLE
Hepatic	HEP	Peritoneum	PER
Brain	BRA	Adrenals	ADR
Lymph nodes	LYM	Skin	SKI
Others	OTH		

R Classification

The absence or presence of residual tumour after treatment may be described by the symbol R. The definitions of the R classification are:

RX   Presence of residual tumour cannot be assessed
R0   No residual tumour
R1   Microscopic residual tumour
R2   Macroscopic residual tumour

Carcinoma of the Skin (excluding eyelid, vulva, and penis) (ICD-O C44.0, 2-9, C63.2)

Rules for Classification

The classification applies only to carcinomas. There should be histological confirmation of the disease and division of cases by histological type.

The following are the procedures for assessing T, N, and M categories:

T categories	Physical examination
N categories	Physical examination and imaging
M categories	Physical examination and imaging

Regional Lymph Nodes

The regional lymph nodes are those appropriate to the site of the primary tumour. See page 112.

TNM Clinical Classification

T – Primary Tumour

TX   Primary tumour cannot be assessed
T0   No evidence of primary tumour
Tis   Carcinoma in situ

T1   Tumour 2 cm or less in greatest dimension
T2   Tumour more than 2 cm but not more than 5 cm in greatest dimension

T3   Tumour more than 5 cm in greatest dimension

T4   Tumour invades deep extradermal structures, i.e., cartilage, skeletal muscle, or bone

Notes: In the case of multiple simultaneous tumours, the tumour with the highest T
category is classified and the number of separate tumours is indicated in
parentheses, e.g., T2(5).

N – Regional Lymph Nodes

NX   Regional lymph nodes cannot be assessed

N0   No regional lymph node metastasis

N1   Regional lymph node metastasis

M – Distant Metastasis

MX   Distant metastasis cannot be assessed

M0   No distant metastasis

M1   Distant metastasis

pTNM Pathological Classification

The pT, pN, and pM categories correspond to the T, N, and M
categories.

pN0 Histological examination of a regional lymphadenectomy specimen will ordinarily include 6 or more lymph nodes.

G Histopathological Grading

GX   Grade of differentiation cannot be assessed

G1   Well differentiated

G2   Moderately differentiated

G3   Poorly differentiated

G4   Undifferentiated

Stage Grouping

Stage 0	Tis	N0	M0
Stage I	T1	N0	M0
Stage II	T2	N0	M0
	T3	N0	M0
Stage III	T4	N0	M0
	Any T	N1	M0
Stage IV	Any T	Any N	M1

Summary

Skin Carcinoma	
T1	≤2 cm
T2	>2 to 5 cm
T3	>5 cm
T4	Deep extradermal structures (cartilage, skeletal muscle, bone)
N1	Regional

Malignant Melanoma of Skin
(ICD-O C44, C51.0, C60.9, C63.2)

Rules for Classification

There should be histological confirmation of the disease.

The following are the procedures for assessing N and M categories:

N categories   Physical examination and imaging
M categories   Physical examination and imaging

Regional Lymph Nodes

The regional lymph nodes are those appropriate to the site of the primary tumour. See page 112.

TNM Clinical Classification

T – Primary Tumour
The extent of the tumour is classified after excision, see pT, page 119.

N – Regional Lymph Nodes
   NX   Regional lymph nodes cannot be assessed
   N0   No regional lymph node metastasis
   N1   Metastasis 3 cm or less in greatest dimension in any regional lymph node(s)

N2   Metastasis more than 3 cm in greatest dimension in any regional lymph node(s) and/or in-transit metastasis

  N2a   Metastasis more than 3 cm in greatest dimension in any regional lymph node(s)

  N2b   In-transit metastasis

  N2c   Both

Note: In-transit metastasis involves skin or subcutaneous tissue more than 2 cm from the primary tumour but not beyond the regional lymph nodes.

M – Distant Metastasis

MX   Distant metastasis cannot be assessed

M0   No distant metastasis

M1   Distant metastasis

  M1a   Metastasis in skin or subcutaneous tissue or lymph node(s) beyond the regional lymph nodes

  M1b   Visceral metastasis

pTNM Pathological Classification

pT – Primary Tumour

pTX   Primary tumour cannot be assessed

pT0   No evidence of primary tumour

pTis   Melanoma in situ (Clark level I) (atypical melanocytic hyperplasia, severe melanocytic dysplasia, not an invasive malignant lesion)

pT1   Tumour 0.75 mm or less in thickness and invades the papillary dermis (Clark level II)

pT2   Tumour more than 0.75 mm but not more than 1.5 mm in thickness and/or invades to the papillary-reticular dermal interface (Clark level III)

pT3   Tumour more than 1.5 mm but not more than 4.0 mm in thickness and/or invades the reticular dermis (Clark level IV)

  pT3a Tumour more than 1.5 mm but not more than
        3.0 mm in thickness
  pT3b Tumour more than 3.0 mm but not more than
        4.0 mm in thickness
pT4 Tumour more than 4.0 mm in thickness and/or
     invades subcutaneous tissue (Clark level V) and/or
     satellite(s) within 2 cm of the primary tumour
  pT4a Tumour more than 4.0 mm in thickness and/or
        invades subcutaneous tissue
  pT4b Satellite(s) within 2 cm of the primary tumour

Note: In case of discrepancy between tumour thickness and level, the pT category is
       based on the less favourable finding.

pN – Regional Lymph Nodes

The pN categories correspond to the N categories.

   pN0 Histological examination of a regional lymphadenectomy specimen will ordinarily include 6 or more lymph nodes.

pM – Distant Metastasis

The pM categories correspond to the M categories.

Stage Grouping

Stage 0	pTis	N0	M0
Stage I	pT1	N0	M0
	pT2	N0	M0
Stage II	pT3	N0	M0
Stage III	pT4	N0	M0
	Any pT	N1, N2	M0
Stage IV	Any pT	Any N	M1

Summary

Skin Malignant Melanoma		
pT1	≤0.75 mm	Level II
pT2	>0.75 to 1.5 mm	Level III
pT3	>1.5 to 4 mm	Level IV
pT4	>4.0 mm/satellites	Level V
N1	Regional <3 cm	
N2	Regional >3 cm and/or in-transit metastasis	

BREAST TUMOURS
(ICD-O C50)

Introductory Notes

The site is described under the following headings:

- Rules for classification with the procedures for assessing T, N, and M categories; additional methods may be used when they enhance the accuracy of appraisal before treatment
- Anatomical subsites
- Definition of the regional lymph nodes
- TNM Clinical classification
- pTNM Pathological classification
- G Histopathological grading
- R Classification
- Stage grouping
- Summary

Rules for Classification

The classification applies only to carcinomas. There should be histological confirmation of the disease. The anatomical subsite of origin should be recorded but is not considered in classification.

In the case of multiple simultaneous primary tumours in one breast, the tumour with the highest T category should be used for classification. Simultaneous *bilateral* breast cancers should be classified independently to permit division of cases by histological type.

The following are the procedures for assessing T, N, and M categories:

T categories	Physical examination and imaging, e.g., mammography
N categories	Physical examination and imaging
M categories	Physical examination and imaging

Anatomical Sites

1. Nipple (C50.0)
2. Central portion (C50.1)
3. Upper-inner quadrant (C50.2)
4. Lower-inner quadrant (C50.3)
5. Upper-outer quadrant (C50.4)
6. Lower-outer quadrant (C50.5)
7. Axillary tail (C50.6)

Regional Lymph Nodes

The regional lymph nodes are:
1. *Axillary* (ipsilateral): interpectoral (Rotter) nodes and lymph nodes along the axillary vein and its tributaries, which may be divided into the following levels:
   (i)   *Level I* (low-axilla): lymph nodes lateral to the lateral border of pectoralis minor muscle.

(ii) *Level II* (mid-axilla): lymph nodes between the medial and lateral borders of the pectoralis minor muscle and the interpectoral (Rotter) lymph nodes.

(iii) *Level III* (apical axilla): lymph nodes medial to the medial margin of the pectoralis minor muscle including those designated as subclavicular, infra-clavicular, or apical.

Note: Intramammary lymph nodes are coded as axillary lymph nodes

2. *Internal mammary* (ipsilateral): lymph nodes in the inter-costal spaces along the edge of the sternum in the endo-thoracic fascia.

Any other lymph node metastasis is coded as a distant metastasis (M1), including supraclavicular, cervical, or con-tralateral internal mammary lymph nodes.

TNM Clinical Classification

T – Primary Tumour

TX   Primary tumour cannot be assessed

T0   No evidence of primary tumour

Tis   Carcinoma in situ: intraductal carcinoma, or lobular carcinoma in situ, or Paget disease of the nipple with no tumour

Note: Paget disease associated with a tumour is classified according to the size of the tumour.

T1   Tumour 2 cm or less in greatest dimension

T1mic Microinvasion 0.1 cm or less in greatest dimension[1]

T1a   More than 0.1 cm but not more than 0.5 cm in greatest dimension

T1b   More than 0.5 cm but not more than 1 cm in greatest dimension

T1c   More than 1 cm but not more than 2 cm in greatest dimension

T2   Tumour more than 2 cm but not more than 5 cm in greatest dimension

T3   Tumour more than 5 cm in greatest dimension

T4   Tumour of any size with direct extension to chest wall or skin

Note: Chest wall includes ribs, intercostal muscles, and serratus anterior muscle but not pectoral muscle

T4a   Extension to chest wall

T4b   Oedema (including peau d'orange), or ulceration of the skin of the breast, or satellite skin nodules confined to the same breast

T4c   Both 4a and 4b, above

T4d   Inflammatory carcinoma[2]

Notes: 1. Microinvasion is the extension of cancer cells beyond the basement membrane into the adjacent tissues with no focus more than 0.1 cm in greatest dimension. When there are multiple foci of microinvasion, the size of only the largest focus is used to classify the microinvasion. (Do not use the sum of all the individual foci.) The presence of multiple foci of microinvasion should be noted, as it is with multiple larger invasive carcinomas.

2. Inflammatory carcinoma of the breast is characterized by diffuse, brawny induration of the skin with an erysipeloid edge, usually with no underlying mass. If the skin biopsy is negative and there is no localized measurable primary cancer, the T category is pTX when pathologically staging a clinical inflammatory carcinoma (T4d). Dimpling of the skin, nipple retraction, or other skin changes, except those in T4b and T4d, may occur in T1, T2, or T3 without affecting the classification.

N – Regional Lymph Nodes

NX   Regional lymph nodes cannot be assessed (e.g., previously removed)

N0   No regional lymph node metastasis

N1   Metastasis to movable ipsilateral axillary node(s)

N2   Metastasis to ipsilateral axillary node(s) fixed to one another or to other structures

N3   Metastasis to ipsilateral internal mammary lymph node(s)

M – Distant Metastasis

MX   Distant metastasis cannot be assessed
M0   No distant metastasis
M1   Distant metastasis

The categories M1 and pM1 may be further specified according to the following notation:

Pulmonary	PUL	Bone marrow	MAR
Osseous	OSS	Pleura	PLE
Hepatic	HEP	Peritoneum	PER
Brain	BRA	Adrenals	ADR
Lymph nodes	LYM	Skin	SKI
Others	OTH		

pTNM Pathological Classification

pT – Primary Tumour

The pathological classification requires the examination of the primary carcinoma with no gross tumour at the margins of resection. A case can be classified pT if there is only microscopic tumour in a margin.

The pT categories correspond to the T categories.

Note: When classifying pT the tumour size is a measurement of the invasive component. If there is a large in situ component (e.g., 4 cm) and a small invasive component (e.g., 0.5 cm), the tumour is coded pT1a.

pN – Regional Lymph Nodes

The pathological classification requires the resection and examination of at least the low axillary lymph nodes (level 1) (see page 124). Such a resection will ordinarily include 6 or more lymph nodes.

pNX Regional lymph nodes cannot be assessed (not removed for study or previously removed)

pN0 No regional lymph node metastasis

pN1 Metastasis to movable ipsilateral axillary node(s)

    pN1a Only micrometastasis (none larger than 0.2 cm)

    pN1b Metastasis to lymph node(s), any larger than 0.2 cm

        pN1bi   Metastasis to 1–3 lymph nodes, any more than 0.2 cm and all less than 2.0 cm in greatest dimension

        pN1bii   Metastasis to 4 or more lymph nodes, any more than 0.2 cm and all less than 2.0 cm in greatest dimension

        pN1biii   Extension of tumour beyond the capsule of a lymph node metastasis less than 2.0 cm in greatest dimension

        pN1biv   Metastasis to a lymph node 2.0 cm or more in greatest dimension

pN2 Metastasis to ipsilateral axillary lymph nodes that are fixed to one another or to other structures

pN3 Metastasis to ipsilateral internal mammary lymph node(s)

pM – Distant Metastasis

The pM categories correspond to the M categories.

G Histopathological Grading

GX Grade of differentiation cannot be assessed

G1 Well differentiated

G2 Moderately differentiated

G3 Poorly differentiated

G4 Undifferentiated

R Classification

The absence or presence of residual tumour after treatment may be described by the symbol R. The definitions of the R classification are:

RX   Presence of residual tumour cannot be assessed
R0   No residual tumour
R1   Microscopic residual tumour
R2   Macroscopic residual tumour

Stage Grouping

Stage 0	Tis	N0	M0
Stage I	T1[1]	N0	M0
Stage IIA	T0	N1	M0
	T1[1]	N1[2]	M0
	T2	N0	M0
Stage IIB	T2	N1	M0
	T3	N0	M0
Stage IIIA	T0	N2	M0
	T1[1]	N2	M0
	T2	N2	M0
	T3	N1, N2	M0
Stage IIIB	T4	Any N	M0
	Any T	N3	M0
Stage IV	Any T	Any N	M1

Notes: 1. T1 includes T1mic
2. The prognosis of patients with pN1a is similar to that of patients with pN0.

Summary

Breast			
Tis	In situ		
T1	≤ 2 cm		
T1mic	≤ 0.1 cm		
T1a	>0.1 to 0.5 cm		
T1b	>0.5 to 1 cm		
T1c	>1 to 2 cm		
T2	>2 to 5 cm		
T3	>5 cm		
T4	Chest wall/skin		
T4a	Chest wall		
T4b	Skin oedema/ulceration, satellite skin nodules		
T4c	Both 4a and 4b		
T4d	Inflammatory carcinoma		
N1	Movable axillary	pN1	
		pN1a	Micrometastasis only, ≤ 0.2 cm

		pN1b	Gross metastasis
			 (i) 1–3 nodes/
			       >0.2 to <2 cm
			 (ii) ≥ 4 nodes/
			       >0.2 to <2 cm
			 (iii) through capsule/
			       <2 cm
			 (iv) ≥ 2 cm

N2	Fixed axillary	pN2	
N3	Internal mammary	pN3	

GYNAECOLOGICAL TUMOURS

Introductory Notes

The following sites are included:

- Vulva
- Vagina
- Cervix uteri
- Corpus uteri
- Ovary
- Fallopian tube
- Gestational trophoblastic tumours

Cervix uteri and corpus uteri were amongst the first sites to be classified by the TNM system. The "League of Nations" stages for carcinoma of the cervix have been used with minor modifications for over 50 years, and, because these are accepted by the Fédération Internationale de Gynécologie et d'Obstétrique (FIGO), the TNM categories have been defined to correspond to the FIGO stages. Some amendments have been made in collaboration with FIGO, and the classifications now published have the approval of the FIGO, UICC, and the national TNM committees including the AJCC.

Each site is described under the following headings:

- Rules for classification with the procedures for assessing T, N, and M categories; additional methods may be used

when they enhance the accuracy of appraisal before treatment
- Anatomical subsites where appropriate
- Definition of the regional lymph nodes
- TNM Clinical classification
- pTNM Pathological classification
- Stage grouping
- Summary

Distant Metastasis

The categories M1 and pM1 may be further specified according to the following notation:

Pulmonary	PUL	Bone marrow	MAR
Osseous	OSS	Pleura	PLE
Hepatic	HEP	Peritoneum	PER
Brain	BRA	Adrenals	ADR
Lymph nodes	LYM	Skin	SKI
Others	OTH		

Histopathological Grading

The definitions of the G categories apply to vulva, vagina, cervix, and fallopian tube. These are:

G – Histopathological Grading

GX Grade of differentiation cannot be assessed
G1 Well differentiated
G2 Moderately differentiated
G3 Poorly differentiated
G4 Undifferentiated

R Classification

The absence or presence of residual tumour after treatment may be described by the symbol R. The definitions of the R classification are:

  RX   Presence of residual tumour cannot be assessed
  R0   No residual tumour
  R1   Microscopic residual tumour
  R2   Macroscopic residual tumour

Vulva
(ICD-O C51)

This classification is in complete agreement with the FIGO classification.

Rules for Classification

The classification applies only to primary carcinomas of the vulva. There should be histological confirmation of the disease.

A carcinoma of the vulva that has extended to the vagina is classified as carcinoma of the vulva.

The following are the procedures for assessing T, N, and M categories:

T categories	Physical examination, endoscopy, and imaging
N categories	Physical examination and imaging
M categories	Physical examination and imaging

The FIGO stages are based on surgical staging. (TNM stages are based on clinical and/or pathological classification.)

Regional Lymph Nodes

The regional lymph nodes are the femoral and inguinal nodes.

TNM Clinical Classification

T – Primary Tumour

TX   Primary tumour cannot be assessed
T0   No evidence of primary tumour
Tis   Carcinoma in situ (preinvasive carcinoma)

T1   Tumour confined to vulva or vulva and perineum, 2 cm or less in greatest dimension
    T1a   Tumour confined to vulva or vulva and perineum, 2 cm or less in greatest dimension and with stromal invasion no greater than 1.0 mm*
    T1b   Tumour confined to vulva or vulva and perineum, 2 cm or less in greatest dimension and with stromal invasion greater than 1.0 mm*
T2   Tumour confined to vulva or vulva and perineum, more than 2 cm in greatest dimension
T3   Tumour invades any of the following: lower urethra, vagina, anus
T4   Tumour invades any of the following: bladder mucosa, rectal mucosa, upper urethral mucosa; or is fixed to pubic bone

Note: *The depth of invasion is defined as the measurement of the tumour from the epithelial-stromal junction of the adjacent most superficial dermal papilla to the deepest point of invasion.

N – Regional Lymph Nodes

NX   Regional lymph nodes cannot be assessed
N0   No regional lymph node metastasis
N1   Unilateral regional lymph node metastasis
N2   Bilateral regional lymph node metastasis

M – Distant Metastasis

MX   Distant metastasis cannot be assessed
M0   No distant metastasis

M1   Distant metastasis (including pelvic lymph node metastasis)

pTNM Pathological Classification

The pT, pN, and pM categories correspond to the T, N, and M categories.

pN0 Histological examination of an inguinal lymphadenectomy specimen will ordinarily include 6 or more lymph nodes.

G Histopathological Grading

See definitions on page 132.

Stage Grouping

Stage 0	Tis	N0	M0
Stage I	T1	N0	M0
Stage IA	T1a	N0	M0
Stage IB	T1b	N0	M0
Stage II	T2	N0	M0
Stage III	T1	N1	M0
	T2	N1	M0
	T3	N0, N1	M0
Stage IVA	T1	N2	M0
	T2	N2	M0
	T3	N2	M0
	T4	Any N	M0
Stage IVB	Any T	Any N	M1

Summary

Vulva	
T1	Confined to vulva/perineum ≤2 cm
T1a	Stromal invasion ≤1.0 mm
T1b	Stromal invasion >1.0 mm
T2	Confined to vulva/perineum >2 cm
T3	Lower urethra/vagina/anus
T4	Bladder mucosa/rectal mucosa/ upper urethral mucosa/bone
N1	Unilateral
N2	Bilateral

Vagina
(ICD-O C52)

The definitions of the T and M categories correspond to the FIGO stages. Both systems are included for comparison.

Rules for Classification

The classification applies to primary carcinomas only.

Tumours present in the vagina as secondary growths from either genital or extragenital sites are excluded.

A tumour that has extended to the portio and reached the external os (orifice of uterus) is classified as carcinoma of the cervix.

A tumour involving the vulva is classified as carcinoma of the vulva.

There should be histological confirmation of the disease.

The following are the procedures for assessing T, N, and M categories:

T categories	Physical examination, endoscopy, and imaging
N categories	Physical examination and imaging
M categories	Physical examination and imaging

Regional Lymph Nodes

Upper two-thirds of vagina: the pelvic nodes
Lower third of vagina: the inguinal nodes

TNM Clinical Classification

T – Primary Tumour

TNM Categories	FIGO Stages	
TX		Primary tumour cannot be assessed
T0		No evidence of primary tumour
Tis	0	Carcinoma in situ (preinvasive carcinoma)
T1	I	Tumour confined to vagina
T2	II	Tumour invades paravaginal tissues but does not extend to pelvic wall
T3	III	Tumour extends to pelvic wall
T4	IVA	Tumour invades *mucosa* of bladder or rectum, and/or extends beyond the true pelvis **Note:** The presence of bullous oedema is not sufficient evidence to classify a tumour as T4.
M1	IVB	Distant metastasis

N – Regional Lymph Nodes

NX Regional lymph nodes cannot be assessed
N0 No regional lymph node metastasis
N1 Regional lymph node metastasis

M – Distant Metastasis

MX Distant metastasis cannot be assessed
M0 No distant metastasis
M1 Distant metastasis

pTNM Pathological Classification

The pT, pN, and pM categories correspond to the T, N, and M categories.

pN0 Histological examination of an inguinal lymphadenectomy specimen will ordinarily include 6 or more lymph nodes; a pelvic lymphadenectomy specimen will ordinarily include 10 or more lymph nodes.

G Histopathological Grading

See definitions on page 132

Stage Grouping

Stage 0	Tis	N0	M0
Stage I	T1	N0	M0
Stage II	T2	N0	M0
Stage III	T1	N1	M0
	T2	N1	M0
	T3	N0, N1	M0
Stage IVA	T4	Any N	M0
Stage IVB	Any T	Any N	M1

Summary

TNM	Vagina	FIGO
T1	Vaginal wall	I
T2	Paravaginal tissue	II
T3	Extends to pelvic wall	III
T4	Mucosa of bladder/rectum, beyond pelvis	IVA
N1	Regional	III
M1	Distant metastasis	IVB

Cervix Uteri
(ICD-O C53)

The definitions of the T and M categories correspond to the FIGO stages. Both systems are included for comparison.

Rules for Classification

The classification applies only to carcinomas. There should be histological confirmation of the disease.

The following are the procedures for assessing T, N, and M categories:

T categories	Physical examination, cystoscopy,* and imaging including urography
N categories	Physical examination and imaging including urography and lymphography
M categories	Physical examination and imaging

Note: *Cystoscopy not required for Tis.

Anatomical Subsites

1. Endocervix (C53.0)
2. Exocervix (C53.1)

Regional Lymph Nodes

The regional lymph nodes are the paracervical, parametrial, hypogastric (internal iliac, obturator), common and external iliac, presacral, and lateral sacral nodes.

TNM Clinical Classification

T – Primary Tumour

TNM Categories	FIGO Stages	
TX		Primary tumour cannot be assessed
T0		No evidence of primary tumour
Tis	0	Carcinoma in situ (preinvasive carcinoma)
T1	I	Cervical carcinoma confined to uterus (extension to corpus should be disregarded)
T1a	IA	Invasive carcinoma diagnosed only by microscopy. All macroscopically visible lesions—even with super-ficial invasion—are T1b/Stage IB
T1a1	IA1	Stromal invasion no greater than 3.0 mm in depth and 7.0 mm or less in horizontal spread
T1a2	IA2	Stromal invasion more than 3.0 mm and not more than 5.0 mm with a horizontal spread 7.0 mm or less
		Note: The depth of invasion should not be more than 5 mm taken from the base of the epithelium, either surface or glandular, from which it origi-nates. The depth of invasion is defined as the measurement of the tumour from the epithelial-stromal junction of the adjacent most superficial epithelial papilla to the deepest point of invasion. Vascular space involvement, venous or lym-phatic, does not affect classification.

TNM Categories	**FIGO Stages**	
T1b	IB	Clinically visible lesion confined to the cervix or microscopic lesion greater than T1a2/IA2
T1b1	IB1	Clinically visible lesion 4.0 cm or less in greatest dimension
T1b2	IB2	Clinically visible lesion more than 4 cm in greatest dimension
T2	II	Tumour invades beyond uterus but not to pelvic wall or to lower third of the vagina
T2a	IIA	Without parametrial invasion
T2b	IIB	With parametrial invasion
T3	III	Tumour extends to pelvic wall and/or involves lower third of vagina and/or causes hydronephrosis or non-functioning kidney
T3a	IIIA	Tumour involves lower third of vagina, no extension to pelvic wall
T3b	IIIB	Tumour extends to pelvic wall and/or causes hydronephrosis or non-functioning kidney
T4	IVA	Tumour invades *mucosa* of bladder or rectum and/or extends beyond true pelvis **Note:** The presence of bullous oedema is not sufficient to classify a tumour as T4.
M1	IVB	Distant metastasis

N – Regional Lymph Nodes

    NX   Regional lymph nodes cannot be assessed
    N0   No regional lymph node metastasis
    N1   Regional lymph node metastasis

M – Distant Metastasis

    MX   Distant metastasis cannot be assessed
    M0   No distant metastasis
    M1   Distant metastasis

pTNM Pathological Classification

The pT, pN, and pM categories correspond to the T, N, and M categories.

pN0 Histological examination of a pelvic lymphadenectomy specimen will ordinarily include 10 or more lymph nodes.

G Histopathological Grading

See definitions on page 132

Stage Grouping

Stage 0	Tis	N0	M0
Stage IA	T1a	N0	M0
Stage IA1	T1a1	N0	M0
Stage IA2	T1a2	N0	M0
Stage IB	T1b	N0	M0
Stage IB1	T1b1	N0	M0
Stage IB2	T1b2	N0	M0
Stage IIA	T2a	N0	M0
Stage IIB	T2b	N0	M0
Stage IIIA	T3a	N0	M0
Stage IIIB	T1	N1	M0
	T2	N1	M0
	T3a	N1	M0
	T3b	Any N	M0
Stage IVA	T4	Any N	M0
Stage IVB	Any T	Any N	M1

Summary

TNM	Cervix Uteri	FIGO
Tis	In situ	0
T1	Confined to uterus	I
T1a	Diagnosed only by microscopy	IA
T1a1	Depth ≤3 mm, horizontal spread ≤7 mm	IA1
T1a2	Depth >3–5 mm, horizontal spread ≤7 mm	IA2
T1b	Clinically visible or microscopic lesion, greater than T1a2	IB
T1b1	≤4 cm	IB1
T1b2	>4 cm	IB2
T2	Beyond uterus but not pelvic wall or lower third vagina	II
T2a	No parametrium	IIA
T2b	Parametrium	IIB
T3	Lower third vagina/pelvic wall/hydronephrosis	III
T3a	Lower third vagina	IIIA
T3b	Pelvic wall/hydronephrosis	IIIB
T4	Mucosa of bladder/rectum; beyond true pelvis	IVA
M1	Distant metastasis	IVB

Corpus Uteri
(ICD-O C54)

The definitions of the T, N, and M categories correspond to the FIGO stages. Both systems are included for comparison.

Rules for Classification

The classification applies only to carcinomas. There should be histological verification and grading of the tumour. The diagnosis should be based on examination of specimens taken by endometrial biopsy.

The following are the procedures for assessing T, N, and M categories:

T categories	Physical examination and imaging including urography and cystoscopy
N categories	Physical examination and imaging including urography
M categories	Physical examination and imaging.

The FIGO stages are based on surgical staging (TNM stages are based on clinical and/or pathological classification).

Anatomical Subsites

1. Isthmus uteri (C54.0)
2. Fundus uteri (C54.3)

Regional Lymph Nodes

The regional lymph nodes are the pelvic (hypogastric [obturator, internal iliac], common and external iliac, parametrial, and sacral) and the para-aortic nodes.

TNM Clinical Classification

T – Primary Tumour

TNM Categories	FIGO Stages	
TX		Primary tumour cannot be assessed
T0		No evidence of primary tumour
Tis	0	Carcinoma in situ (preinvasive carcinoma)
T1	I	Tumour confined to corpus uteri
T1a	IA	Tumour limited to endometrium
T1b	IB	Tumour invades up to less than one half of myometrium
T1c	IC	Tumour invades to more than one half of myometrium
T2	II	Tumour invades cervix but does not extend beyond uterus
T2a	IIA	Endocervical glandular involvement only
T2b	IIB	Cervical stromal invasion
T3 and/or N1	III	Local and/or regional spread as specified in T3a, b, N1, and FIGO IIIA, B, C below
T3a	IIIA	Tumour involves serosa and/or adnexa (direct extension or metastasis) and/or cancer cells in ascites or peritoneal washings
T3b	IIIB	Vaginal involvement (direct extension or metastasis)
N1	IIIC	Metastasis to pelvic and/or para-aortic lymph nodes

TNM Categories	**FIGO stages**	
T4	IVA	Tumour invades bladder *mucosa* and/or bowel *mucosa*
		Note: The presence of bullous edema is not sufficient evidence to classify a tumour as T4.
M1	IVB	Distant metastasis (*excluding* metastasis to vagina, pelvic serosa, or adnexa, *including* metastasis to intra-abdominal lymph nodes other than para-aortic and/or inguinal nodes)

N – Regional Lymph Nodes

NX   Regional lymph nodes cannot be assessed
N0   No regional lymph node metastasis
N1   Regional lymph node metastasis

M – Distant Metastasis

MX   Distant metastasis cannot be assessed
M0   No distant metastasis
M1   Distant metastasis

pTNM Pathological Classification

The pT, pN, and pM categories correspond to the T, N, and M categories.

pN0 Histological examination of a pelvic lymphadenectomy specimen will ordinarily include 10 or more lymph nodes.

G Histopathological Grading

For histopathological grading see the following publications:

FIGO (1989) Annual report on the results of treatment in gynecological cancer. Int J Gynecol Obstet 28: 189–193

FIGO (1990) Changes in gynecological cancer staging by the International Federation of Gynecology and Obstetrics. Am J Obstet Gynecol 162: 610–611

Stage Grouping

Stage 0	Tis	N0	M0
Stage IA	T1a	N0	M0
Stage IB	T1b	N0	M0
Stage IC	T1c	N0	M0
Stage IIA	T2a	N0	M0
Stage IIB	T2b	N0	M0
Stage IIIA	T3a	N0	M0
Stage IIIB	T3b	N0	M0
Stage IIIC	T1	N1	M0
	T2	N1	M0
	T3a, b	N1	M0
Stage IVA	T4	Any N	M0
Stage IVB	Any T	Any N	M1

Summary

TNM	Corpus Uteri	FIGO
Tis	In situ	0
T1	Confined to corpus	I
T1a	Tumour limited to the endometrium	IA
T1b	Up to less than half of myometrium	IB
T1c	More than half of myometrium	IC
T2	Extension to cervix	II
T2a	Endocervical glandular only	IIA
T2b	Cervical stroma	IIB
T3 and/or N1	Local and/or regional as specified below	III
T3a	Serosa/adnexa/positive peritoneal cytology	IIIA
T3b	Vaginal involvement	IIIB
N1	Regional lymph node metastasis	IIIC
T4	Mucosa of bladder/bowel	IVA
M1	Distant metastasis	IVB

Ovary
(ICD-O C56)

The definitions of the T, N, and M categories correspond to the FIGO stages. Both systems are included for comparison.

Rules for Classification

There should be histological confirmation of the disease and division of cases by histological type. In accordance with FIGO, a simplified version of the WHO histological classification of common epithelial tumours (1973) is recommended. The degree of differentiation (grade) should be recorded.

The following are the procedures for assessing T, N, and M categories:

T categories	Physical examination, imaging, laparoscopy, and/or surgical exploration
N categories	Physical examination, imaging, laparoscopy, and/or surgical exploration
M categories	Physical examination, imaging, laparoscopy, and/or surgical exploration

Regional Lymph Nodes

The regional lymph nodes are the hypogastric (obturator), common iliac, external iliac, lateral sacral, para-aortic, and inguinal nodes.

TNM Clinical Classification

T – Primary Tumour

TNM Categories	FIGO Stages	
TX		Primary tumour cannot be assessed
T0		No evidence of primary tumour
T1	I	Tumour limited to the ovaries
T1a	IA	Tumour limited to one ovary; capsule intact, no tumour on ovarian surface; no malignant cells in ascites or peritoneal washings
T1b	IB	Tumour limited to both ovaries; capsule intact, no tumour on ovarian surface; no malignant cells in ascites or peritoneal washings
T1c	IC	Tumour limited to one or both ovaries with any of the following: capsule ruptured, tumour on ovarian surface, malignant cells in ascites or peritoneal washings
T2	II	Tumour involves one or both ovaries with pelvic extension
T2a	IIA	Extension and/or implants on uterus and/or tube(s); no malignant cells in ascites or peritoneal washings
T2b	IIB	Extension to other pelvic tissues; no malignant cells in ascites or peritoneal washings
T2c	IIC	Pelvic extension (2a or 2b) with malignant cells in ascites or peritoneal washings

TNM Categories	FIGO Stages	
T3 and/or N1	III	Tumour involves one or both ovaries with microscopically confirmed peritoneal metastasis outside the pelvis and/or regional lymph node metastasis
T3a	IIIA	Microscopic peritoneal metastasis beyond pelvis
T3b	IIIB	Macroscopic peritoneal metastasis beyond pelvis 2 cm or less in greatest dimension
T3c and/ or N1	IIIC	Peritoneal metastasis beyond pelvis more than 2 cm in greatest dimension and/or regional lymph node metastasis
M1	IV	Distant metastasis (excludes peritoneal metastasis)

Note: Liver capsule metastasis is T3/stage III, liver parenchymal metastasis M1/stage IV. Pleural effusion must have positive cytology for M1/stage IV.

N – Regional Lymph Nodes

NX   Regional lymph nodes cannot be assessed
N0   No regional lymph node metastasis
N1   Regional lymph node metastasis

M – Distant Metastasis

MX   Distant metastasis cannot be assessed
M0   No distant metastasis
M1   Distant metastasis

pTNM Pathological Classification

The pT, pN, and pM categories correspond to the T, N, and M categories.

pN0 Histological examination of a pelvic lymphadenectomy specimen will ordinarily include 10 or more lymph nodes.

G Histopathological Grading

GX	Grade cannot be assessed
GB	Borderline malignancy
G1	Well differentiated
G2	Moderately differentiated
G3–4	Poorly differentiated or undifferentiated

Stage Grouping

Stage IA	T1a	N0	M0
Stage IB	T1b	N0	M0
Stage IC	T1c	N0	M0
Stage IIA	T2a	N0	M0
Stage IIB	T2b	N0	M0
Stage IIC	T2c	N0	M0
Stage IIIA	T3a	N0	M0
Stage IIIB	T3b	N0	M0
Stage IIIC	T3c	N0	M0
	Any T	N1	M0
Stage IV	Any T	Any N	M1

Summary

TNM	Ovary	FIGO
T1	Limited to the ovaries	I
T1a	One ovary, capsule intact	IA
T1b	Both ovaries, capsule intact	IB
T1c	Capsule ruptured, tumour on surface, malignant cells in ascites or peritoneal washings	IC
T2	Pelvic extension	II
T2a	Uterus, tube(s)	IIA
T2b	Other pelvic tissues	IIB
T2c	Malignant cells in ascites or peritoneal washings	IIC
T3 and/or N1	Peritoneal metastasis beyond pelvis and/or regional lymph node metastasis	III
T3a	Microscopic peritoneal metastasis	IIIA
T3b	Macroscopic peritoneal metastasis ≤ 2 cm	IIIB
T3c and/or N1	Peritoneal metastasis >2 cm and/or regional lymph node metastasis	IIIC
M1	Distant metastasis (excludes peritoneal metastasis)	IV

Fallopian Tube
(ICD-O C57.0)

The following classification for carcinoma of the fallopian tube is based on that of FIGO adopted in 1992. The definitions of the T, N, and M categories correspond to the FIGO stages. Both systems are included for comparison.

Rules for Classification

The classification applies only to carcinoma. There should be histological confirmation of the disease.
   The following are the procedures for assessing T, N, and M categories:

T categories	Physical examination, imaging, laparoscopy, and/or surgical exploration
N categories	Physical examination, imaging, laparoscopy, and/or surgical exploration
M categories	Physical examination, imaging, laparoscopy, and/or surgical exploration

The FIGO stages are based on surgical staging. (TNM stages are based on clinical and/or pathological staging).

Regional Lymph Nodes

The regional lymph nodes are the hypogastric (obturator), common iliac, external iliac, lateral sacral, para-aortic, and inguinal nodes.

TNM Clinical Classification

T – Primary Tumour

TNM Categories	FIGO Stages	
TX		Primary tumour cannot be assessed
T0		No evidence of primary tumour
Tis	0	Carcinoma in situ (preinvasive carcinoma)
T1	I	Tumour confined to fallopian tube(s)
T1a	IA	Tumour limited to one tube, without penetrating the serosal surface; no ascites
T1b	IB	Tumour limited to both tubes, without penetrating the serosal surface; no ascites
T1c	IC	Tumour limited to one or both tube(s) with extension onto or through the tubal serosa, or with malignant cells in ascites or peritoneal washings
T2	II	Tumour involves one or both fallopian tube(s) with pelvic extension
T2a	IIA	Extension and/or metastasis to uterus and/or ovaries
T2b	IIB	Extension to other pelvic structures
T2c	IIC	Pelvic extension (2a or 2b) with malignant cells in ascites or peritoneal washings

TNM Categories	FIGO Stages	
T3 and/or N1	III	Tumour involves one or both fallopian tube(s) with peritoneal implants outside the pelvis and/or positive regional lymph nodes
T3a	IIIA	Microscopic peritoneal metastasis outside the pelvis
T3b	IIIB	Macroscopic peritoneal metastasis outside the pelvis 2 cm or less in greatest dimension
T3c and/or N1	IIIC	Peritoneal metastasis more than 2 cm in greatest dimension and/or positive regional lymph nodes
M1	IV	Distant metastasis (excludes peritoneal metastasis)

N – Regional Lymph Nodes

NX   Regional lymph nodes cannot be assessed
N0   No regional lymph node metastasis
N1   Regional lymph node metastasis

M – Distant Metastasis

MX   Distant metastasis cannot be assessed
M0   No distant metastasis
MX   Distant metastasis

pTNM Pathological Classification

The pT, pN, and pM categories correspond to the T, N, and M categories.

pN0 Histological examination of a pelvic lymphadenectomy specimen will ordinarily include 10 or more lymph nodes.

G Histopathological Grading

See definitions on page 132.

Stage Grouping

Stage 0	Tis	N0	M0
Stage IA	T1a	N0	M0
Stage IB	T1b	N0	M0
Stage IC	T1c	N0	M0
Stage IIA	T2a	N0	M0
Stage IIB	T2b	N0	M0
Stage IIC	T2c	N0	M0
Stage IIIA	T3a	N0	M0
Stage IIIB	T3b	N0	M0
Stage IIIC	T3c	N0	M0
	Any T	N1	M0
Stage IV	Any T	Any N	M1

Summary

TNM	Fallopian Tube	FIGO
T1	Limited to tube(s)	I
T1a	One tube; serosa intact	IA
T1b	Both tubes; serosa intact	IB
T1c	Serosa penetrated, malignant cells in ascites or peritoneal washings	IC
T2	Pelvic extension	II
T2a	Uterus and/or ovaries	IIA
T2b	Other pelvic structures	IIB
T2c	Malignant cells in ascites or peritoneal washings	IIC
T3 and/or N1	Peritoneal metastasis outside the pelvis and/or regional lymph node metastasis	III
T3a	Microscopic peritoneal metastasis	IIIA
T3b	Macroscopic peritoneal metastasis ≤ 2 cm	IIIB
T3 and/or N1	Peritoneal metastasis >2 cm and/or regional lymph node metastasis	IIIC
M1	Distant metastasis (excludes peritoneal metastasis)	IV

Gestational Trophoblastic Tumours
(ICD-O C58.9)

The following classification for gestational trophoblastic tumours is based on that of FIGO adopted 1992. The definitions of T and M categories correspond to the FIGO stages. Both systems are included for comparison. In stage grouping, risk factors are considered in addition to T and M. In contrast to other sites, an N (regional lymph node) classification does not apply to these tumours.

Rules for Classification

The classification applies to choriocarcinoma (9100/3), invasive hydatidiform mole (9100/1), and placental site trophoblastic tumour (9104/1). Placental site tumours should be reported separately. Histological confirmation is not required if the urine human chorionic gonadotropin (hCG) level is abnormally elevated. History of prior chemotherapy for this disease should be noted.

The following are the procedures for assessing T and M categories:

T categories:	Physical examination, imaging including urography and cystoscopy, and urine hCG level
M categories:	Physical examination, imaging, and assessment of urine hCG level
Risk factors:	There are two major risk factors that may affect outcome (other than T and M):
	1. hCG more than 100,000 IU/24 h urine
	2. Detection of disease longer than 6 months from termination of antecedent pregnancy

TM Clinical Classification

T–Primary Tumour

TM Categories	FIGO Stages*	
TX		Primary tumour cannot be assessed
T0		No evidence of primary tumour
T1	I	Tumour confined to uterus
T2	II	Tumour extends to other genital structures: vagina, ovary, broad ligament, fallopian tube by metastasis or direct extension
M1a	III	Metastasis to the lung(s)
M1b	IV	Other distant metastasis with or without lung involvement

Note: *Stages I to IV are subdivided into A to C according to the number of risk factors:

A without risk factors
B with one risk factor
C with two risk factors

M – Metastasis

MX Metastasis cannot be assessed
M0 No distant metastasis
M1 Distant metastasis
M1a Metastasis to lung(s)
M1b Other distant metastasis with or without lung involvement

Note: Genital metastasis (vagina, ovary, broad ligament, fallopian tube) is classified T2.

pTM Pathological Classification

The pT and pM categories correspond to the T and M categories.

Stage Grouping

Stage	T	M	Risk Factors
IA	T1	M0	without
IB	T1	M0	one
IC	T1	M0	two
IIA	T2	M0	without
IIB	T2	M0	one
IIC	T2	M0	two
IIIA	Any T	M1a	without
IIIB	Any T	M1a	one
IIIC	Any T	M1a	two
IVA	Any T	M1b	without
IVB	Any T	M1b	one
IVC	Any T	M1b	two

Summary

TM	Gestational Trophoblastic Tumours	Stage
T1	Confined to uterus	I
T2	Other genital structures	II
M1a	Metastasis to lung(s)	III
M1b	Other distant metastasis	IV
	Risk factors: • hCG >100,000 IU/24 h urine • detection of disease >6 months from pregnancy	Stages are subdivided: A without risk factors B with one risk factor C with two risk factors

UROLOGICAL TUMOURS

Introductory Notes

The following sites are included:

- Penis
- Prostate
- Testis
- Kidney
- Renal pelvis and ureter
- Urinary bladder
- Urethra

Each site is described under the following headings:

- Rules for classification with the procedures for assessing T, N, and M categories; additional methods may be used when they enhance the accuracy of appraisal before treatment
- Anatomical sites and subsites where appropriate
- Definition of the regional lymph nodes
- Distant metastasis
- TNM Clinical classification
- pTNM Pathological classification
- G Histopathological grading where applicable
- Stage grouping
- Summary

Distant Metastasis

The categories M1 and pM1 may be further specified according to the following notation:

Pulmonary	PUL	Bone marrow	MAR
Osseous	OSS	Pleura	PLE
Hepatic	HEP	Peritoneum	PER
Brain	BRA	Adrenals	ADR
Lymph nodes	LYM	Skin	SKI
Others	OTH		

R Classification

The absence or presence of residual tumour after treatment may be described by the symbol R. The definitions of the R classification are:

RX   Presence of residual tumour cannot be assessed
R0   No residual tumour
R1   Microscopic residual tumour
R2   Macroscopic residual tumour

Penis
(ICD-O C60)

Rules for Classification

The classification applies only to carcinomas. There should be histological confirmation of the disease.

The following are the procedures for assessing T, N, and M categories:

T categories	Physical examination and endoscopy
N categories	Physical examination and imaging
M categories	Physical examination and imaging

Anatomical Subsites

1. Prepuce (C60.0)
2. Glans penis (C60.1)
3. Shaft of penis (C60.2)

Regional Lymph Nodes

The regional lymph nodes are the superficial and deep inguinal and the pelvic nodes.

TNM Clinical Classification

T – Primary Tumour

TX	Primary tumour cannot be assessed
T0	No evidence of primary tumour
Tis	Carcinoma in situ
Ta	Noninvasive verrucous carcinoma

T1   Tumour invades subepithelial connective tissue
T2   Tumour invades corpus spongiosum or cavernosum
T3   Tumour invades urethra or prostate
T4   Tumour invades other adjacent structures

N – Regional Lymph Nodes

NX   Regional lymph nodes cannot be assessed
N0   No regional lymph node metastasis
N1   Metastasis in a single superficial inguinal lymph node
N2   Metastasis in multiple or bilateral superficial inguinal lymph nodes
N3   Metastasis in deep inguinal or pelvic lymph node(s), unilateral or bilateral

M – Distant Metastasis

MX   Distant metastasis cannot be assessed
M0   No distant metastasis
M1   Distant metastasis

pTNM Pathological Classification

The pT, pN, and pM categories correspond to the T, N, and M categories.

G Histopathological Grading

GX   Grade of differentiation cannot be assessed
G1   Well differentiated
G2   Moderately differentiated
G3–4   Poorly differentiated/undifferentiated

Stage Grouping

Stage 0	Tis	N0	M0
	Ta	N0	M0
Stage I	T1	N0	M0
Stage II	T1	N1	M0
	T2	N0, N1	M0
Stage III	T1	N2	M0
	T2	N2	M0
	T3	N0, N1, N2	M0
Stage IV	T4	Any N	M0
	Any T	N3	M0
	Any T	Any N	M1

Summary

Penis	
Tis	In situ
Ta	Noninvasive verrucous carcinoma
T1	Subepithelial connective tissue
T2	Corpus spongiosum, cavernosum
T3	Urethra, prostate
T4	Other adjacent structures
N1	One superficial inguinal
N2	Multiple or bilateral superficial inguinal
N3	Deep inguinal or pelvic

Prostate
(ICD-O C61)

Rules for Classification

The classification applies only to adenocarcinomas. Transitional cell carcinoma of the prostate is classified as a urethral tumour (see page 191). There should be histological confirmation of the disease.

The following are the procedures for assessing T, N, and M categories:

T categories	Physical examination, imaging, endoscopy, biopsy, and biochemical tests
N categories	Physical examination and imaging
M categories	Physical examination, imaging, skeletal studies, and biochemical tests

Regional Lymph Nodes

The regional lymph nodes are the nodes of the true pelvis, which essentially are the pelvic nodes below the bifurcation of the common iliac arteries. Laterality does not affect the N classification.

TNM Clinical Classification

T – Primary Tumour

TX   Primary tumour cannot be assessed
T0   No evidence of primary tumour

T1　Clinically inapparent tumour not palpable or visible by imaging

　　T1a　Tumour incidental histological finding in 5% or less of tissue resected

　　T1b　Tumour incidental histological finding in more than 5% of tissue resected

　　T1c　Tumour identified by needle biopsy (e.g., because of elevated PSA)

T2　Tumour confined within the prostate[1]

　　T2a　Tumour involves one lobe

　　T2b　Tumour involves both lobes

T3　Tumour extends through the prostatic capsule[2]

　　T3a　Extracapsular extension (unilateral or bilateral)

　　T3b　Tumour invades seminal vesicle(s)

T4　Tumour is fixed or invades adjacent structures other than seminal vesicles: bladder neck, external sphincter, rectum, levator muscles, and/or pelvic wall

Notes: 1. Tumour found in one or both lobes by needle biopsy, but not palpable or visible by imaging, is classified as T1c.
2. Invasion into the prostatic apex or into (but not beyond) the prostatic capsule is not classified as T3, but as T2.

N – Regional Lymph Nodes

NX　Regional lymph nodes cannot be assessed

N0　No regional lymph node metastasis

N1　Regional lymph node metastasis

M – Distant Metastasis

MX　Distant metastasis cannot be assessed

M0　No distant metastasis

M1　Distant metastasis

　　M1a　Non-regional lymph node(s)

　　M1b　Bone(s)

　　M1c　Other site(s)

Note: When more than one site of metastasis is present, the most advanced category should be used.

pTNM Pathological Classification

The pT, pN, and pM categories correspond to the T, N, and M categories.

However, there is no pT1 category because there is insufficient tissue to assess the highest pT category.

G Histopathological Grading

GX   Grade cannot be assessed
G1   Well differentiated (slight anaplasia)
G2   Moderately differentiated (moderate anaplasia)
G3–4 Poorly differentiated/undifferentiated (marked anaplasia)

Stage Grouping

Stage I	T1a	N0	M0	G1
Stage II	T1a	N0	M0	G2, 3–4
	T1b	N0	M0	Any G
	T1c	N0	M0	Any G
	T1	N0	M0	Any G
	T2	N0	M0	Any G
Stage III	T3	N0	M0	Any G
Stage IV	T4	N0	M0	Any G
	Any T	N1	M0	Any G
	Any T	Any N	M1	Any G

Summary

Prostate	
T1	Not palpable or visible
T1a	≤5%
T1b	>5%
T1c	Needle biopsy
T2	Confined within prostate
T2a	One lobe
T2b	Both lobes
T3	Through prostatic capsule
T3a	Extracapsular
T3b	Seminal vesicle(s)
T4	Fixed or invades adjacent structures: bladder neck, external sphincter, rectum, levator muscles, pelvic wall
N1	Regional lymph node(s)
M1a	Non-regional lymph node(s)
M1b	Bone(s)
M1c	Other site(s)

Testis
(ICD-O C62)

Rules for Classification

The classification applies only to germ cell tumours of the testis. There should be histological confirmation of the disease and division of cases by histological type. Histopathological grading is not applicable.

The presence of elevated serum tumour markers, including alphafetoprotein (AFP), human chorionic gonadotropin (hCG), and lactate dehydrogenase (LDH), is frequent in this disease. Staging is based on the determination of the anatomic extent of disease and assessment of serum tumour markers.

The following are the procedures for assessing N, M, and S categories:

N categories	Physical examination and imaging
M categories	Physical examination, imaging, and biochemical tests
S categories	Serum tumour markers

Stages are subdivided based on the presence and degree of elevation of serum tumour markers. Serum tumour markers are obtained immediately after orchiectomy and, if elevated, should be performed serially after orchiectomy according to the normal decay for AFP (half-life 7days) and hCG (half-life 3 days) to assess for serum tumour marker elevation. The S classification is based on the nadir value of hCG and AFP after orchiectomy. The serum level of LDH (but not its half-life levels) has prognostic value in patients with metastatic disease and is included for staging.

Regional Lymph Nodes

The regional lymph nodes are the abdominal para-aortic (periaortic), preaortic, interaortocaval, precaval, paracaval, retrocaval, and retroaortic nodes. Nodes along the spermatic vein should be considered regional. Laterality does not affect the N classification. The intrapelvic nodes and the inguinal nodes are considered regional after scrotal or inguinal surgery.

TNM Clinical Classification

T – Primary tumour

The extent of the primary tumour is classified after radical orchiectomy; see pT. If no radical orchiectomy has been performed, TX is used.

N – Regional Lymph Nodes
NX   Regional lymph nodes cannot be assessed
N0   No regional lymph node metastasis
N1   Metastasis with a lymph node mass 2 cm or less in greatest dimension or multiple lymph nodes, none more than 2 cm in greatest dimension
N2   Metastasis with a lymph node mass more than 2 cm but not more than 5 cm in greatest dimension, or multiple lymph nodes, any one mass more than 2 cm but not more than 5 cm in greatest dimension
N3   Metastasis with a lymph node mass more than 5 cm in greatest dimension

M – Distant Metastasis
MX   Distant metastasis cannot be assessed
M0   No distant metastasis

M1   Distant metastasis
  M1a   Non-regional lymph node or pulmonary metastasis
  M1b   Distant metastasis other than to non-regional lymph nodes and lungs

pTNM Pathological Classification

pT – Primary Tumour

pTX   Primary tumour cannot be assessed (if no radical orchiectomy has been performed TX is used)
pT0   No evidence of primary tumour (e.g. histologic scar in testis)
pTis   Intratubular germ cell neoplasia (carcinoma in situ)

pT1   Tumour limited to testis and epididymis without vascular/lymphatic invasion; tumour may invade tunica albuginea but not tunica vaginalis.
pT2   Tumour limited to testis and epididymis with vascular/lymphatic invasion, or tumour extending through tunica albuginea with involvement of tunica vaginalis.
pT3   Tumour invades spermatic cord with or without vascular/lymphatic invasion.
pT4   Tumour invades scrotum with or without vascular/lymphatic invasion.

pN – Regional Lymph Nodes

pNX   Regional lymph nodes cannot be assessed
pN0   No regional lymph node metastasis
pN1   Metastasis with a lymph node mass 2 cm or less in greatest dimension and 5 or fewer positive nodes, none more than 2 cm in greatest dimension
pN2   Metastasis with a lymph node mass more than 2 cm but not more than 5 cm in greatest dimension; or more

than 5 nodes positive, none more than 5 cm; or evidence of extranodal extension of tumour
pN3 Metastasis with a lymph node mass more than 5 cm in greatest dimension

pM – Distant Metastasis

The pM category corresponds to the M category.

S – Serum Tumour Markers

SX Serum marker studies not available or not performed
S0 Serum marker study levels within normal limits

	LDH		**hCG (mIU/ml)**		**AFP (ng/ml)**
S1	$<1.5 \times N$	and	$<5{,}000$	and	$<1{,}000$
S2	$1.5–10 \times N$	or	$5{,}000–50{,}000$	or	$1{,}000–10{,}000$
S3	$>10 \times N$	or	$>50{,}000$	or	$>10{,}000$

N indicates the upper limit of normal for the LDH assay

Stage Grouping

Stage 0	pTis	N0	M0	S0,SX
Stage I	pT1–4	N0	M0	SX
Stage IA	pT1	N0	M0	S0
Stage IB	pT2	N0	M0	S0
	pT3	N0	M0	S0
	pT4	N0	M0	S0
Stage IS	Any pT/TX	N0	M0	S1–3
Stage II	Any pT/TX	N1–3	M0	SX
Stage IIA	Any pT/TX	N1	M0	S0
	Any pT/TX	N1	M0	S1
Stage IIB	Any pT/TX	N2	M0	S0
	Any pT/TX	N2	M0	S1
Stage IIC	Any pT/TX	N3	M0	S0
	Any pT/TX	N3	M0	S1
Stage III	Any pT/TX	Any N	M1, M1a	SX
Stage IIIA	Any pT/TX	Any N	M1, M1a	S0
	Any pT/TX	Any N	M1, M1a	S1
Stage IIIB	Any pT/TX	N1–3	M0	S2
	Any pT/TX	Any N	M1, M1a	S2
Stage IIIC	Any pT/TX	N1–3	M0	S3
	Any pT/TX	Any N	M1, M1a	S3
	Any pT/TX	Any N	M1b	Any S

Summary

Testis	
pTis	Intratubular
pT1	Testis and epididymis, no vascular/lymphatic invasion
pT2	Testis and epididymis with vascular/lymphatic invasion or tunica vaginalis
pT3	Spermatic cord
pT4	Scrotum
N1	≤2 cm
N2	>2 to 5 cm
N3	>5 cm
M1a	Non-regional lymph node or pulmonary metastasis
M1b	Non-pulmonary visceral metastasis

Kidney
(ICD-O C64)

Rules for Classification

The classification applies only to renal cell carcinoma. There should be histological confirmation of the disease.

The following are the procedures for assessing T, N, and M categories:

T categories   Physical examination and imaging
N categories   Physical examination and imaging
M categories   Physical examination and imaging

Regional Lymph Nodes

The regional lymph nodes are the hilar, abdominal para-aortic, and paracaval nodes. Laterality does not affect the N categories.

TNM Clinical Classification

T – Primary Tumour

TX   Primary tumour cannot be assessed
T0   No evidence of primary tumour
T1   Tumour 7.0 cm or less in greatest dimension, limited to the kidney
T2   Tumour more than 7.0 cm in greatest dimension, limited to the kidney

T3   Tumour extends into major veins or invades adrenal
      gland or perinephric tissues but not beyond Gerota
      fascia
      T3a   Tumour invades adrenal gland or perinephric
             tissues but not beyond Gerota fascia
      T3b   Tumour grossly extends into renal vein(s) or
             vena cava below diaphragm
      T3c   Tumour grossly extends into vena cava above
             diaphragm
T4   Tumour invades beyond Gerota fascia

N – Regional Lymph Nodes

NX   Regional lymph nodes cannot be assessed
N0   No regional lymph node metastasis
N1   Metastasis in a single regional lymph node
N2   Metastasis in more than one regional lymph node

M – Distant Metastasis

MX   Distant metastasis cannot be assessed
M0   No distant metastasis
M1   Distant metastasis

pTNM Pathological Classification

The pT, pN, and pM categories correspond to the T, N, and M
categories.

G Histopathological Grading

GX   Grade of differentiation cannot be assessed
G1   Well differentiated
G2   Moderately differentiated
G3–4   Poorly differentiated/undifferentiated

Stage Grouping

Stage I	T1	N0	M0
Stage II	T2	N0	M0
Stage III	T1	N1	M0
	T2	N1	M0
	T3	N0, N1	M0
Stage IV	T4	N0, N1	M0
	Any T	N2	M0
	Any T	Any N	M1

Summary

Kidney	
T1	≤7.0 cm; limited to the kidney
T2	>7.0 cm; limited to the kidney
T3	Into major veins; adrenal or perinephric invasion
T4	Invades beyond Gerota fascia
N1	Single
N2	More than one

Renal Pelvis and Ureter
(ICD-O C65, C66)

Rules for Classification

The classification applies only to carcinomas. Papilloma is excluded. There should be histological or cytological confirmation of the disease.

The following are the procedures for assessing T, N, and M categories:

T categories	Physical examination, imaging, and endoscopy
N categories	Physical examination and imaging
M categories	Physical examination and imaging

Anatomical Sites

1. Renal pelvis (C65)
2. Ureter (C66)

Regional Lymph Nodes

The regional lymph nodes are the hilar, abdominal para-aortic, and paracaval nodes and, for ureter, intrapelvic nodes. Laterality does not affect the N classification.

TNM Clinical Classification

T – Primary Tumour

TX   Primary tumour cannot be assessed
T0   No evidence of primary tumour
Ta   Noninvasive papillary carcinoma
Tis Carcinoma in situ

T1   Tumour invades subepithelial connective tissue
T2   Tumour invades muscularis
T3   *(Renal pelvis)* Tumour invades beyond muscularis into peripelvic fat or renal parenchyma
     (Ureter) Tumour invades beyond muscularis into periureteric fat
T4   Tumour invades adjacent organs or through the kidney into perinephric fat

N – Regional Lymph Nodes

NX   Regional lymph nodes cannot be assessed
N0   No regional lymph node metastasis
N1   Metastasis in a single lymph node 2 cm or less in greatest dimension
N2   Metastasis in a single lymph node more than 2 cm but not more than 5 cm in greatest dimension, or multiple lymph nodes, none more than 5 cm in greatest dimension
N3   Metastasis in a lymph node more than 5 cm in greatest dimension

M – Distant Metastasis

MX   Distant metastasis cannot be assessed
M0   No distant metastasis
M1   Distant metastasis

pTNM Pathological Classification

The pT, pN, and pM categories correspond to the T, N, and M categories.

G Histopathological Grading

GX	Grade of differentiation cannot be assessed
G1	Well differentiated
G2	Moderately differentiated
G3–4	Poorly differentiated/undifferentiated

Stage Grouping

Stage 0a	Ta	N0	M0
0is	Tis	N0	M0
Stage I	T1	N0	M0
Stage II	T2	N0	M0
Stage III	T3	N0	M0
Stage IV	T4	N0	M0
	Any T	N1, N2, N3	M0
	Any T	any N	M1

Summary

Renal Pelvis, Ureter	
Ta	Noninvasive papillary
Tis	In situ
T1	Subepithelial connective tissue
T2	Muscularis
T3	Beyond muscularis
T4	Adjacent organs, perinephric fat
N1	Single ≤2 cm
N2	Single >2 to 5 cm, multiple ≤5 cm
N3	>5 cm

Urinary Bladder
(ICD-O C67)

Rules for Classification

The classification applies only to carcinomas. Papilloma is excluded. There should be histological or cytological confirmation of the disease.

The following are the procedures for assessing T, N, and M categories:

T categories	Physical examination, imaging, and endoscopy
N categories	Physical examination and imaging
M categories	Physical examination and imaging

Regional Lymph Nodes

The regional lymph nodes are the nodes of the true pelvis, which essentially are the pelvic nodes below the bifurcation of the common iliac arteries. Laterality does not affect the N classification.

TNM Clinical Classification

T – Primary Tumour

The suffix (m) should be added to the appropriate T category to indicate multiple tumours. The suffix (is) may be added to any T to indicate presence of associated carcinoma in situ.

TX   Primary tumour cannot be assessed
T0   No evidence of primary tumour
Ta   Noninvasive papillary carcinoma
Tis   Carcinoma in situ: "flat tumour"

T1   Tumour invades subepithelial connective tissue
T2   Tumour invades muscle
      T2a   Tumour invades superficial muscle (inner half)
      T2b   Tumour invades deep muscle (outer half)
T3   Tumour invades perivesical tissue:
      T3a   microscopically
      T3b   macroscopically (extravesical mass)
T4   Tumour invades any of the following: prostate, uterus, vagina, pelvic wall, abdominal wall
      T4a   Tumour invades prostate or uterus or vagina
      T4b   Tumour invades pelvic wall or abdominal wall

N – Regional Lymph Nodes

NX   Regional lymph nodes cannot be assessed
N0   No regional lymph node metastasis
N1   Metastasis in a single lymph node 2 cm or less in greatest dimension
N2   Metastasis in a single lymph node more than 2 cm but not more than 5 cm in greatest dimension, or multiple lymph nodes, none more than 5 cm in greatest dimension
N3   Metastasis in a lymph node more than 5 cm in greatest dimension

M – Distant Metastasis

MX   Distant metastasis cannot be assessed
M0   No distant metastasis
M1   Distant metastasis

pTNM Pathological Classification

The pT, pN, and pM categories correspond to the T, N, and M categories.

G Histopathological Grading

GX   Grade of differentiation cannot be assessed
G1   Well differentiated
G2   Moderately differentiated
G3–4   Poorly differentiated/undifferentiated

Stage Grouping

Stage 0a	Ta	N0	M0
Stage 0is	Tis	N0	M0
Stage I	T1	N0	M0
Stage II	T2a	N0	M0
	T2b	N0	M0
Stage III	T3a	N0	M0
	T3b	N0	M0
	T4a	N0	M0
Stage IV	T4b	N0	M0
	Any T	N1, 2, 3	M0
	Any T	Any N	M1

Summary

Urinary Bladder	
Ta	Noninvasive papillary
Tis	In situ: "flat tumour"
T1	Subepithelial connective tissue
T2	Muscularis
T2a	Inner half
T2b	Outer half
T3	Beyond muscularis
T3a	Microscopically
T3b	Extravesical mass
T4a	Prostate, uterus, vagina
T4b	Pelvic wall, abdominal wall
N1	Single ≤2 cm
N2	Single >2 to 5cm, multiple ≤5 cm
N3	>5 cm

Urethra

Rules for Classification

The classification applies to carcinomas of the urethra (ICD-O C68.0) and transitional cell carcinomas of the prostate (ICD-O C61) and prostatic urethra. There should be histological or cytological confirmation of the disease.

The following are the procedures for assessing T, N, and M categories:

T categories	Physical examination, imaging, and endoscopy
N categories	Physical examination and imaging
M categories	Physical examination and imaging

Regional Lymph Nodes

The regional lymph nodes are the inguinal and the pelvic nodes. Laterality does not affect the N classification.

TNM Clinical Classification

T – Primary Tumour

TX   Primary tumour cannot be assessed
T0   No evidence of primary tumour

Urethra (male and female)
Ta   Noninvasive papillary, polypoid, or verrucous carcinoma
Tis   Carcinoma in situ

T1   Tumour invades subepithelial connective tissue

T2   Tumour invades any of the following: corpus spongi-
      osum, prostate, periurethral muscle

T3   Tumour invades any of the following: corpus caver-
      nosum, beyond prostatic capsule, anterior vagina,
      bladder neck

T4   Tumour invades other adjacent organs

Transitional cell carcinoma of prostate (prostatic urethra)

Tis pu   Carcinoma in situ, involvement of prostatic urethra

Tis pd   Carcinoma in situ, involvement of prostatic ducts

T1   Tumour invades subepithelial connective tissue

T2   Tumour invades any of the following: prostatic stroma,
      corpus spongiosum, periurethral muscle

T3   Tumour invades any of the following: corpus caver-
      nosum, beyond prostatic capsule, bladder neck (extra-
      prostatic extension)

T4   Tumour invades other adjacent organs (invasion of
      the bladder)

N – Regional Lymph Nodes

NX   Regional lymph nodes cannot be assessed

N0   No regional lymph node metastasis

N1   Metastasis in a single lymph node 2 cm or less in
      greatest dimension

N2   Metastasis in a single lymph node more than 2 cm in
      greatest dimension, or multiple lymph nodes

M – Distant Metastasis

MX   Distant metastasis cannot be assessed

M0   No distant metastasis

M1   Distant metastasis

pTNM Pathological Classification

The pT, pN, and pM categories correspond to the T, N, and M categories.

G Histopathological Grading

GX	Grade of differentiation cannot be assessed
G1	Well differentiated
G2	Moderately differentiated
G3–4	Poorly differentiated/undifferentiated

Stage Grouping

Stage 0a	Ta	N0	M0
0is	Tis	N0	M0
	Tis pu	N0	M0
	Tis pd	N0	M0
Stage I	T1	N0	M0
Stage II	T2	N0	M0
Stage III	T1	N1	M0
	T2	N1	M0
	T3	N0, N1	M0
Stage IV	T4	N0, N1	M0
	Any T	N2	M0
	Any T	Any N	M1

Summary

Urethra	
Ta	Noninvasive papillary, polypoid, or verrucous
Tis	In situ
T1	Subepithelial connective tissue
T2	Corpus spongiosum, prostate, periurethral muscle
T3	Corpus cavernosum, beyond prostatic capsule, anterior vagina, bladder neck
T4	Other adjacent organs
N1	Single ≤2 cm
N2	>2 cm or multiple

Transitional Cell Carcinoma of Prostate (Prostatic Urethra)	
Tis pu	In situ, prostatic urethra
Tis pd	In situ, prostatic ducts
T1	Subepithelial connective tissue
T2	Prostatic stroma, corpus spongiosum, periurethral muscle
T3	Corpus cavernosum, beyond prostatic capsule, bladder neck (extraprostatic extension)
T4	Other adjacent organs (bladder)

OPHTHALMIC TUMOURS

Introductory Notes

Tumours of the eye and its adnexa are a disparate group including carcinoma, melanoma, sarcomas, and retinoblastoma. For clinical convenience they are classified in one section.

The following sites are included:

- Eyclid (eyelid melanoma is classified with skin tumours)
- Conjunctiva
- Uvea
- Retina
- Orbit
- Lacrimal gland

For histological nomenclature and diagnostic critcria, reference to the WHO classification (Zimmerman, LE: Histological typing of tumours of the eye and its adnexa. WHO, Geneva 1980) is recommended.

Each tumour type is described under the following headings:

- Rules for classification with the proccdures for assessing the T, N, and M categories
- Anatomical sites where appropriate
- Definition of the regional lymph nodes
- TNM Clinical classification

- pTNM Pathological classification
- G Histopathological grading where applicable
- Stage grouping where applicable
- Summary

Regional Lymph Nodes

The definitions of N categories for ophthalmic tumours are:

N – Regional Lymph Nodes

NX   Regional lymph nodes cannot be assessed
N0   No regional lymph node metastasis
N1   Regional lymph node metastasis

Distant Metastasis

The definitions of the M categories for ophthalmic tumours are:

M – Distant Metastasis

MX   Distant metastasis cannot be assessed
M0   No distant metastasis
M1   Distant metastasis

The categories M1 and pM1 may be further specified according to the following notation:

Pulmonary	PUL	Bone marrow	MAR
Osseous	OSS	Pleura	PLE
Hepatic	HEP	Peritoneum	PER
Brain	BRA	Adrenals	ADR
Lymph nodes	LYM	Skin	SKI
Others	OTH		

Histopathological Grading

The following definitions of the G categories apply to carcinoma of the eyelid and conjunctiva and sarcoma of the orbit. These are:

G – Histopathological Grading
GX   Grade of differentiation cannot be assessed
G1   Well differentiated
G2   Moderately differentiated
G3   Poorly differentiated
G4   Undifferentiated

R Classification

The absence or presence of residual tumour after treatment may be described by the symbol R. The definitions of the R classification apply to all ophthalmic tumours. These are:

RX   Presence of residual tumour cannot be assessed
R0   No residual tumour
R1   Microscopic residual tumour
R2   Macroscopic residual tumour

Carcinoma of Eyelid
(ICD-O C44.1)

Rules of Classification

There should be histological confirmation of the disease and division of cases by histological type, e.g., basal cell, squamous cell, sebaceous carcinoma. Melanoma of the eyelid is classified with skin tumours, see page 118.

The following are procedures for assessing T, N, and M categories:

T categories	Physical examination
N categories	Physical examination
M categories	Physical examination and imaging

Regional Lymph Nodes

The regional lymph nodes are the preauricular, submandibular and cervical lymph nodes.

TNM Clinical Classification

T – Primary Tumour

TX   Primary tumour cannot be assessed
T0   No evidence of primary tumour
Tis   Carcinoma in situ

T1   Tumour of any size, not invading the tarsal plate; or at eyelid margin, 5 mm or less in greatest dimension

T2   Tumour invades tarsal plate; or at eyelid margin, more than 5 mm but not more than 10 mm in greatest dimension

T3   Tumour involves full eyelid thickness; or at eyelid margin, more than 10 mm in greatest dimension

T4   Tumour invades adjacent structures

N – Regional Lymph Nodes

See definitions on page 196.

M – Distant Metastasis

See definitions on page 196.

pTNM Pathological Classification

The pT, pN, and pM categories correspond to the T, N, and M categories.

G Histopathological Grading

See definitions on page 197.

Stage Grouping

No stage grouping is at present recommended.

Summary

Eyelid Carcinoma	
T1	Not in tarsal plate Lid margin: ≤5 mm
T2	In tarsal plate Lid margin: >5 to 10 mm
T3	Full thickness Lid margin: >10 mm
T4	Adjacent structures
N1	Regional

Carcinoma of Conjunctiva
(ICD-O C 69.0)

Rules for Classification

There should be histological confirmation of the disease and division of cases by histological type, e.g., mucoepidermoid and squamous cell carcinoma.

The following are the procedures for assessing T, N, and M categories:

T categories	Physical examination
N categories	Physical examination
M categories	Physical examination and imaging

Regional Lymph Nodes

The regional lymph nodes are the preauricular, submandibular and cervical lymph nodes.

TNM Clinical Classification

T – Primary Tumour

TX   Primary tumour cannot be assessed
T0   No evidence of primary tumour
Tis   Carcinoma in situ

T1   Tumour 5 mm or less in greatest dimension
T2   Tumour more than 5 mm in greatest dimension, without invasion of adjacent structures
T3   Tumour invades adjacent structures, excluding the orbit
T4   Tumour invades the orbit

N – Regional Lymph Nodes

See definitions on page 196.

M – Distant Metastasis

See definitions on page 196.

pTNM Pathological Classification

The pT, pN, and pM categories correspond to the T, N, and M categories.

G Histopathological Grading

See definitions on page 197.

Stage Grouping

No stage grouping is at present recommended.

Summary

Conjunctiva Carcinoma	
T1	≤5 mm
T2	>5 mm without invasion of adjacent structures
T3	Adjacent structures
T4	Orbit
N1	Regional

Malignant Melanoma of Conjunctiva (ICD-O C69.0)

Rules for Classification

The classification applies only to malignant melanoma.

There should be histological confirmation of the disease. The tumour should be distinguished from non-tumourous pigmentation.

The following are the procedures for assessing T, N, and M categories:

T categories	Physical examination
N categories	Physical examination
M categories	Physical examination and imaging

Regional Lymph Nodes

The regional lymph nodes are the preauricular, submandibular and cervical lymph nodes.

TNM Clinical Classification

T – Primary Tumour
- TX   Primary tumour cannot be assessed
- T0   No evidence of primary tumour

- T1   Tumour(s) of bulbar conjunctiva occupying one quadrant or less

T2   Tumour(s) of bulbar conjunctiva occupying more than one quadrant
T3   Tumour(s) of conjunctival fornix and/or palpebral conjunctiva and/or caruncle
T4   Tumour invades eyelid, cornea, and/or orbit

N – Regional Lymph Nodes
See definitions on page 196.

M – Distant Metastasis
See definitions on page 196.

pTNM Pathological Classification

pT – Primary Tumour
pTX   Primary tumour cannot be assessed
pT0   No evidence of primary tumour

pT1   Tumour(s) of bulbar conjunctiva occupying one quadrant or less and 2 mm or less in thickness
pT2   Tumour(s) of bulbar conjunctiva occupying more than one quadrant and 2 mm or less in thickness
pT3   Tumour(s) of conjunctival fornix and/or palpebral conjunctiva and/or caruncle or tumour of bulbar conjunctiva more than 2 mm in thickness
pT4   Tumour invades eyelid, cornea, and/or orbit

pN – Regional Lymph Nodes
The pN categories correspond to the N categories.

pM – Distant Metastasis
The pM categories correspond to the M categories.

G Histopathological Grading

GX   Grade cannot be assessed
G0   Primary acquired melanosis
G1   Malignant melanoma arising from a naevus
G2   Malignant melanoma arising from primary acquired melanosis
G3   Malignant melanoma arising de novo

Stage Grouping

No stage grouping is at present recommended.

Summary

Malignant Melanoma of Conjunctiva			
T1	Bulbar conjunctiva ≤1 quadrant	pT1	T1 ≤2 mm thick
T2	Bulbar conjunctiva >1 quadrant	pT2	T2 <2 mm thick
T3	Fornix, palpebral conjuntiva, caruncle	pT3	T1 or T2 >2 mm thick and/or T3
T4	Invasion of eyelid, cornea, and/or orbit	pT4	T4
N1	Regional	pN1	Regional

Malignant Melanoma of Uvea
(ICD-O C69.3,4)

Rules for Classification

There should be histological confirmation of the disease.

The following are the procedures for assessing T, N, and M categories:

T categories	Physical examination; additional methods such as fluorescein angiography and isotope examination may enhance the accuracy of appraisal
N categories	Physical examination
M categories	Physical examination and imaging

Regional Lymph Nodes

The regional lymph nodes are the preauricular, submandibular, and cervical nodes.

Anatomical Sites

1. Iris (C69.4)
2. Ciliary body (C69.4)
3. Choroid (C69.3)

TNM Clinical Classification

T – Primary Tumour

TX   Primary tumour cannot be assessed
T0   No evidence of primary tumour

Iris
T1   Tumour limited to the iris
T2   Tumour involves one quadrant or less, with invasion into anterior chamber angle
T3   Tumour involves more than one quadrant, with invasion into anterior chamber angle, ciliary body, and/or choroid
T4   Tumour with extraocular extension

Ciliary Body
T1   Tumour limited to the ciliary body
T2   Tumour invades anterior chamber and/or iris
T3   Tumour invades choroid
T4   Tumour with extraocular extension

Choroid
T1   Tumour 10 mm or less in greatest dimension with an elevation 3 mm or less*
    T1a   Tumour 7 mm or less in greatest dimension with an elevation 2 mm or less
    T1b   Tumour more than 7 mm but not more than 10 mm in greatest dimension with an elevation more than 2 mm but not more than 3 mm
T2   Tumour more than 10 mm but not more than 15 mm in greatest dimension with an elevation more than 3 mm but not more than 5 mm*
T3   Tumour more than 15 mm in greatest dimension or with an elevation more than 5 mm*
T4   Tumour with extraocular extension

Note: *When dimension and elevation show a difference in classification, the highest category should be used for classification. The tumour base may be estimated in optic disc diameters (dd, average 1 dd = 1.5 mm) and the elevation in dioptres (average 3 dioptres = 1 mm); other techniques, such as ultrasonography and computerized stereometry, may provide a more accurate measurement.

N – Regional Lymph Nodes

See definitions on page 196.

M – Distant Metastasis

See definitions on page 196.

pTNM Pathological Classification

The pT, pN, and pM categories correspond to the T, N, and M categories.

G Histopathological Grading

- GX Grade cannot be assessed
- G1 Spindle cell melanoma
- G2 Mixed cell melanoma
- G3 Epithelioid cell melanoma

V Venous Invasion

- VX Venous invasion cannot be assessed
- V0 Veins do not contain tumour
- V1 Veins in melanoma contain tumour
- V2 Vortex veins contain tumour

S Scleral Invasion

- SX Scleral invasion cannot be assessed
- S0 Sclera does not contain tumour
- S1 Intrascleral* invasion of tumour
- S2 Extrascleral invasion of tumour

Note: *Includes perineural and perivascular tumour invasion of scleral canals.

Stage Grouping

If more than one of the uveal structures is involved, the classification of the most affected structure should be used.

Iris and Ciliary Body

Stage I	T1	N0	M0
Stage II	T2	N0	M0
Stage III	T3	N0	M0
Stage IVA	T4	N0	M0
Stage IVB	Any T	N1	M0
	Any T	Any N	M1

Choroid

Stage IA	T1a	N0	M0
Stage IB	T1b	N0	M0
Stage II	T2	N0	M0
Stage III	T3	N0	M0
Stage IVA	T4	N0	M0
Stage IVB	Any T	N1	M0
	Any T	Any N	M1

Summary

Uvea Malignant Melanoma	
	Iris Malignant Melanoma
T1	Iris
T2	≤1 quadrant with invasion into chamber angle
T3	>1 quadrant with invasion into chamber angle, ciliary body, and/or choroid
T4	Extraocular extension
	Ciliary Body Malignant Melanoma
T1	Ciliary body
T2	Anterior chamber and/or iris
T3	Choroid
T4	Extraocular extension
	Choroid Malignant Melanoma
T1	≤10 mm greatest dimension, ≤3 mm elevation
T1a	≤7 mm greatest dimension, ≤2 mm elevation
T1b	>7 to 10 mm greatest dimension, >2 to 3 mm elevation
T2	>10 to 15 greatest dimension, >3 to 5 mm elevation
T3	>15 mm greatest dimension or >5 mm elevation
T4	Extraocular extension
	All Sites
N1	Regional

Retinoblastoma
(ICD-O C69.2)

Rules for Classification

In bilateral cases, the eyes should be classified separately. The classification does not apply to complete spontaneous regression of the tumour. There should be histological confirmation of the disease in an enucleated eye.

The following are the procedures for assessing T, N, and M categories:

T categories	Physical examination and imaging
N categories	Physical examination
M categories	Physical examination and imaging; examination of bone marrow and cerebrospinal fluid may enhance the accuracy of appraisal

Regional Lymph Nodes

The regional lymph nodes are the preauricular, submandibular, and cervical lymph nodes.

TNM Clinical Classification

The extent of retinal involvement is indicated as a percentage.

T – Primary Tumour

TX   Primary tumour cannot be assessed
T0   No evidence of primary tumour

T1   Tumour(s) limited to 25% of the retina or less
T2   Tumour(s) involve(s) more than 25% but not more than 50% of retina
T3   Tumour(s) involve(s) more than 50% of the retina and/or invade(s) beyond the retina but remain(s) intraocular

    T3a   Tumour(s) involve(s) more than 50% of the retina and/or tumour cells in the vitreous body

    T3b   Tumour(s) involve(s) optic disc

    T3c   Tumour(s) involve(s) anterior chamber and/or uvea

T4   Tumour with extraocular invasion

    T4a   Tumour invades retrobulbar optic nerve

    T4b   Extraocular extension other than invasion of optic nerve

Note: The following suffixes may be added to the appropriate T categories:

    (m)   to indicate multiple tumours, e.g., T2(m)
    (f)   to indicate cases with a known family history
    (d)   to indicate diffuse retinal involvement without the formation of discrete masses

N – Regional Lymph Nodes

See definitions on page 196.

M – Distant Metastasis

See definitions on page 196.

pTNM Pathological Classification

pT – Primary Tumour

pTX   Primary tumour cannot be assessed
pT0   No evidence of primary tumour

pT1   Corresponds to T1
pT2   Corresponds to T2
pT3   Corresponds to T3
    pT3a   Corresponds to T3a
    pT3b   Tumour invades optic nerve as far as lamina cribrosa
    pT3c   Tumour in anterior chamber and/or invasion with thickening of uvea and/or intrascleral invasion
pT4   Corresponds to T4
    pT4a   Intraneural tumour beyond lamina cribosa, but not at line of resection
    pT4b   Tumour at line of resection or other extraocular extension

pN – Regional Lymph Nodes

The pN categories correspond to the N categories.

pM – Distant Metastasis

The pM categories correspond to the M categories.

Stage Grouping

Stage IA	T1	N0	M0
Stage IB	T2	N0	M0
Stage IIA	T3a	N0	M0
Stage IIB	T3b	N0	M0
Stage IIC	T3c	N0	M0
Stage IIIA	T4a	N0	M0
Stage IIIB	T4b	N0	M0
Stage IV	Any T	N1	M0
	Any T	Any N	M1

Summary

Retinoblastoma				
T1/pT1	≤25% of retina			
T2/pT2	>25% to 50% of retina			
T3/pT3	>50% of retina and/or intraocular beyond retina			
T3a/pT3a	>50% of retina and/or cells in vitreous			
T3b	Optic disc	pT3b	Optic nerve up to lamina cribrosa	
T3c	Anterior chamber and/or uvea	pT3c	Anterior chamber and/or uvea and/or intrascleral	
T4/pT4	Extraocular			
T4a	Optic nerve	pT4a	Beyond lamina cribrosa, not at resection line	
T4b	Other extraocular	pT4b	Other extraocular and/or at resection line	
N1/pN1	Regional			

Sarcoma of Orbit
(ICD-O C69.6)

Rules for Classification

The classification applies only to sarcomas of soft tissue and bone.

There should be histological confirmation of the disease and division of cases by histological type.

The following are the procedures for assessing T, N, and M categories:

T categories	Physical examination and imaging
N categories	Physical examination
M categories	Physical examination and imaging

Regional Lymph Nodes

The regional lymph nodes are the preauricular, submandibular, and cervical lymph nodes.

TNM Clinical Classification

T – Primary Tumour

TX   Primary tumour cannot be assessed
T0   No evidence of primary tumour

T1   Tumour 15 mm or less in greatest dimension
T2   Tumour more than 15 mm in greatest dimension
T3   Tumour of any size with diffuse invasion of orbital tissues and/or bony walls
T4   Tumour invades beyond the orbit to adjacent sinuses and/or to cranium

N – Regional Lymph Nodes

See definitions on page 196.

M – Distant Metastasis

See definitions on page 196.

pTNM Pathological Classification

The pT, pN, and pM categories correspond to the T, N, and M categories.

G Histopathological Grading

See definitions on page 197.

   Histopathological grading of the tumour should be reported and may have an effect on the staging of these tumours.

Stage Grouping

No stage grouping is at present recommended.

Summary

Sarcoma of Orbit	
T1	≤15 mm
T2	>15 mm
T3	Invades orbital tissues/bony walls
T4	Invades beyond orbit
N1	Regional

Carcinoma of Lacrimal Gland
(ICD-O C69.5)

Rules for Classification

There should be histological confirmation of the disease and division of cases by histological type.

The following are the procedures for assessing T, N, and M categories:

T categories	Physical examination and imaging
N categories	Physical examination
M categories	Physical examination and imaging

Regional Lymph Nodes

The regional lymph nodes are the preauricular, submandibular, and cervical lymph nodes.

TNM Clinical Classification

T – Primary Tumour

TX   Primary tumour cannot be assessed
T0   No evidence of primary tumour

T1   Tumour 2.5 cm or less in greatest dimension, limited to the lacrimal gland
T2   Tumour 2.5 cm or less in greatest dimension, invading the periosteum of the fossa of the lacrimal gland

T3   Tumour more than 2.5 cm but not more than 5 cm in
      greatest dimension
      T3a   Tumour limited to the lacrimal gland
      T3b   Tumour invades the periosteum of the fossa of
             the lacrimal gland
T4   Tumour more than 5 cm in greatest dimension
      T4a   Tumour invades orbital soft tissues, optic
             nerve, or globe, but *without* bone invasion.
      T4b   Tumour invades orbital soft tissues, optic
             nerve, or globe, *with* bone invasion

N – Regional Lymph Nodes

See definitions on page 196.

M – Distant Metastasis

See definitions on page 196.

pTNM Pathological Classification

The pT, pN, and pM categories correspond to the T, N, and M
categories.

G Histopathological Grading

GX   Grade of differentiation cannot be assessed
G1   Well differentiated
G2   Moderately differentiated; includes adenoid cystic
      carcinoma without basaloid (solid) pattern
G3   Poorly differentiated; includes adenoid cystic carci-
      noma with basaloid (solid) pattern
G4   Undifferentiated

Stage Grouping

No stage grouping is at present recommended.

Summary

Lacrimal Gland Carcinoma	
T1	≤2.5 cm, limited to gland
T2	≤2.5 cm, periosteum
T3	>2.5 to 5 cm
T3a	Limited to gland
T3b	Periosteum
T4	>5 cm
T4a	Orbit but not orbital bone
T4b	Orbit and orbital bone
N1	Regional

HODGKIN DISEASE

Introductory Notes

At the present time it is not considered practical to propose a TNM classification for Hodgkin disease.

Following the development of the Ann Arbor classification for Hodgkin disease in 1971, the significance of two important observations with major impact on staging has been appreciated. First, extralymphatic disease, if localized and related to adjacent lymph node disease, does not adversely affect the survival of patients. Secondly, laparotomy with splenectomy has been introduced as a method of obtaining more information on the extent of the disease within the abdomen.

A stage classification based on information from histopathological examination of the spleen and lymph nodes obtained at laparotomy cannot be compared with another without such exploration. Therefore, two systems of classification are presented, a clinical (cS) and a pathological (pS).

Clinical Staging (cS)

Although recognized as incomplete, this is easily performed and should be reproducible from one centre to another. It is determined by history, clinical examination, imaging, blood analysis, and the initial biopsy report. Bone marrow biopsy must be taken from a clinically or radiologically non-involved area of bone.

Liver Involvement

Clinical evidence of liver involvement must include either enlargement of the liver and at least an abnormal serum alkaline phosphatase level and two different liver function test abnormalities, or an abnormal liver demonstrated by imaging and one abnormal liver function test.

Spleen Involvement

Clinical evidence of spleen involvement is accepted if there is palpable enlargement of the spleen confirmed by imaging.

Lymphatic and Extralymphatic Disease

The lymphatic structures are as follows:

- Lymph nodes
- Waldeyer ring
- Spleen
- Appendix
- Thymus
- Peyer patches

The lymph nodes are grouped into regions and one or more (2, 3, etc.) may be involved. The spleen is designated S and extralymphatic organs or sites E.

Lung Involvement

Lung involvement limited to one lobe, or perihilar extension associated with ipsilateral lymphadenopathy, or unilateral pleural effusion with or without lung involvement but with hilar lymphadenopathy is considered as **localized** extralymphatic disease.

Liver Involvement

Liver involvement is always considered as **diffuse** extralymphatic disease.

Pathological Staging (pS)

This takes into account additional data and has a higher degree of precision. It should be applied whenever possible. A – (minus) or + (plus) sign should be added to the various symbols for the examined tissues, depending on the results of histopathological examination.

Histopathological Information

This is classified by symbols indicating the tissue sampled. The following notation is common to the distant metastases (or M1 categories) of all regions classified by the TNM system. However, in order to conform with the Ann Arbor classification, the initial letters used in that system are also given.

Pulmonary	PUL or L	Bone marrow	MAR or M
Osseous	OSS or O	Pleura	PLE or P
Hepatic	HEP or H	Peritoneum	PER
Brain	BRA	Adrenals	ADR
Lymph nodes	LYM or N	Skin	SKI or D
Others	OTH		

Clinical Stages (cS)

Stage I   Involvement of a single lymph node region (I), or localized involvement of a single extralymphatic organ or site (I_E)

Stage II   Involvement of two or more lymph node regions on the same side of the diaphragm (II), or localized involvement of a single extralymphatic organ or site and its regional lymph node(s) with or without involvement of other lymph node regions on the same side of the diaphragm (II_E)

Note: The number of lymph node regions involved may be indicated by a subscript (e.g. II_3)

Stage III   Involvement of lymph node regions on both sides of the diaphragm (III), which may also be accompanied by localized involvement of an associated extralymphatic organ or site (III_E), or by involvement of the spleen (III_S), or both (III_{E+S})

Stage IV   Disseminated (multifocal) involvement of one or more extralymphatic organs, with or without associated lymph node involvement; or isolated extralymphatic organ involvement with distant (non-regional) nodal involvement

Note: The site of Stage IV disease is identified further by specifying sites according to the notations listed above.

A and B Classification (Symptoms)

Each stage should be divided into A and B according to the absence or presence of defined general symptoms. These are:

1. Unexplained weight loss of more than 10% of the usual body weight in the 6 months prior to first attendance
2. Unexplained fever with temperature above 38° C
3. Night sweats

Note: Pruritus alone does not qualify for B classification nor does a short, febrile illness associated with a known infection.

Pathological Stages (pS)

The definitions of the four stages follow the same criteria as the clinical stages but with the additional information obtained following laparotomy. Splenectomy, liver biopsy, lymph node biopsy, and marrow biopsy are mandatory for the establishment of pathological stages. The results of these biopsies are recorded as indicated above (see pages 223 and 224).

Summary

Stage	Hodgkin Disease	Substage
Stage I	Single node region Localized single extralymphatic organ/site	I_E
Stage II	Two or more node regions, same side of diaphragm Localized single extralymphatic organ/ site with its regional nodes, $\pm$ other node regions same side of diaphragm	II_E
Stage III	Node regions both sides of diaphragm $\pm$ Localized single extralymphatic organ/site Spleen Both	III_E III_S III_{E+S}
Stage IV	Diffuse or multifocal involvement of extralymphatic organ(s) $\pm$ regional nodes; isolated extralymphatic organ and non-regional nodes	
All stages divided	Without weight loss/fever/sweats With weight loss/fever/sweats	A B

NON-HODGKIN LYMPHOMAS

As in Hodgkin disease, at the present time it is not considered practical to propose a TNM classification for non-Hodgkin lymphomas. Since no other convincing and tested staging system is available, the Ann Arbor classification is recommended with the same modification as for Hodgkin disease (see page 221).